MORE PRAISE FOR *CARE WORK*

"I'm overjoyed that artists and activists like Leah are writing books like this one that helps water the roots of Disability Justice. This book is coming from the bed, the streets, and on stages where Leah has spoke, taught, performed, and struggled on—that's why it's so accessible and brings lived knowledge into our outdated, stiff institutions and activist movements. In this era of hyper-capitalism, toxic hyper-masculinity, and White supremacy, we desperately need *Care Work*."

—Leroy F. Moore Jr., cofounder of Sins Invalid, cofounder of
National Black Disability Coalition

"*Care Work* is a necessary intervention for those in queer/trans people-of-color spaces and white disability spaces alike, but more importantly, it's an offering of love to all of us living at multiple margins, between spaces of recognition and erasure, who desperately need what Leah has to say. This book is an invitation to dream and to build and to love, as slowly and imperfectly and unevenly as we need to."

—Lydia X. Z. Brown, coeditor of *All the Weight of Our Dreams:*
On Living Racialized Autism

"We have mad crip dreams. In those dreams there exists a decolonized, liberated future in which none of our bodies and lives are disposable. Leah reminds us that turning these dreams into radical practices has already been done, is happening right now within disability justice movements, and will continue to build a future where we are all free. This book is a touchstone for our journey."

—Qwo-Li Driskill, author of *Asegi Stories:*
Cherokee Queer and Two-Spi

LEAH LAKSHMI PIEPZNA-SAMARASINHA

CARE WORK

DREAMING DISABILITY JUSTICE

ARSENAL PULP PRESS
Suite 202 – 211 East Georgia St.
Vancouver, BC V6A 1Z6
Canada
arsenalpulp.com

The publisher gratefully acknowledges the support of the Canada Council for the Arts and the
British Columbia Arts Council for its publishing program, and the Government of Canada, and the
Government of British Columbia (through the Book Publishing Tax Credit Program), for its publishing
activities.

  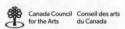 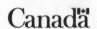

Arsenal Pulp Press acknowledges the xʷməθkʷəy̓əm (Musqueam), Sḵwx̱wú7mesh (Squamish), and
səlilwətaɬ (Tsleil-Waututh) Nations, custodians of the traditional, ancestral, and unceded territories
where our office is located. We pay respect to their histories, traditions, and continuous living cultures
and commit to accountability, respectful relations, and friendship.

Cover and text design by Oliver McPartlin
Cover illustration by TextaQueen
Edited by Lisa Factora-Borchers
Copy edited by Shirarose Wilensky
Proofread by Alison Strobel

Printed and bound in Canada

Library and Archives Canada Cataloguing in Publication:
Piepzna-Samarasinha, Leah Lakshmi, 1975–, author
        Care work : dreaming disability justice / Leah Lakshmi Piepzna-Samarasinha.
Issued in print and electronic formats.
ISBN 978-1-55152-738-3 (softcover).—ISBN 978-1-55152-739-0 (HTML)
        1. People with disabilities. 2. Social justice. I. Title.
HV1568.P54 2018   362.4   C2018-901956-5
                                                               C2018-901957-3

I have loved disabled people of color my whole adult
life and am still amazed to discover that the more I love
our people, the more I remember where I come from.
I remember that my ancestors found each other out,
seeing each other in the unseen. My ancestors knew
that asking after one another and making sure folks had
what they need (what we might understand as collective
access) was the only way to be together; together, the
best shot at staying alive. My ancestors knew the power
of vulnerability and how to hold each other in dignity.
My ancestors knew joy. My ancestors made mistakes and
meditated on who they wanted to be in community.
My ancestors became those people.
—Stacey Milbern

To the beloved, kindred, needed

CONTENTS

IV

THANKS AND ACKNOWLEDGMENTS

This book was written in the matrix of many sick and disabled femme of color care webs, in unceded and occupied Tkaronto/Dish With One Spoon territories, Ohlone territories (Oakland, California), and my current home in South Seattle on Duwamish territories governed by the Treaty of Point Elliot, as well as on a lot of planes, trains, and Megabuses. No matter where I was paying rent, these pieces were mostly written in the majestic disabled revolutionary space of writing from my bed in old sleep pants. So thank you to this decolonial, queer, disabled bed space of wild disabled femme of color dreams.

This book is also emphatically not the product of a single smart and special person's brain. It was made through many community conversations, organizing efforts, arguments, fuckups, terrible challenges and Crazy brilliant ideas and leaps of faith. These ideas were crafted by collective disabled genius, science, and labor. I am not the one right kind of cripple, the kind that is convenient enough to nod at and ignore all the rest. I am all the rest.

So: thank you beyond measure to all the people who have collectively made the disability justice movement and communities, in meetings and at kitchen tables, in femmecaves and online. Thank you to Sins Invalid, disabled, sick, mad, and Deaf communities in Toronto, Oakland, Seattle, and beyond, the Sick and Disabled Queers, Autistic Queer/Trans People of Color, and SDQTPOC Facebook groups, the Deaf Poets Society, the Canaries, Harriet Tubman Collective, Krip-Hop Nation, Performance/Disability/Art (PDA), QPOCirus, Autistic Hoya, Disability Justice Collective Seattle, and GaySL. To cane and chair dancing circles in Toronto and beyond. To everyone who has participated and helped create the Frida and Harriet's Children writing classes online. To the disabled femme artists and organizers, Black, brown, and working class, who mentored and mothered me as a young disabled femme of color writer and taught me how to steal office supplies, get grant money, and find jobs that left me time and spoons to write—Lilith Finkler, Nalo Hopkinson, Elizabeth Ruth, and Patty Berne. Rest in power, Nicole Demerin.

There are many comrades and friends I owe my life and also the thinking and writing in this book to, and here are some: Stacey Milbern, Neve Kamilah Mazique-Bianco, Billie Rain, Lydia X. Z. Brown, Patty Berne, Leroy Moore, Jonah Aline Daniel, Qwo-Li Driskill, Aurora Levins Morales, Cyree Jarelle Johnson, Maria Palacios, Carolyn Lazard, Naima Niambi Lowe, Syrus Marcus Ware, Elena Rose, Meg Day, Elliott Fukui, Aaron Ambrose, Mia Mingus, Shayda Kaftal, Dolores Tejada, Setareh Mohammed, Luci Marie Powers, Aruna Zehra, Amirah Mizrahi, Adrian Nation, Aishah Amatullah, Inbar Frishman, Carrie Martha, Kai Cheng Thom, Lumpen Rolletariat, Gesig Selena Isaac, Loree Erickson, E.T. Russian, Ejeris Dixon, Liz Latty, Zavisha Chromicz, S.B. McKenna, Amalle Dublon, Tina Zavitsanos, you are the best friends for this journey, and I love being on it with you. Thank you to Lisa Amin and Chanelle Gallant for being my oldest sisters. To autistic and neurodivergent communities for welcoming me home.

Thank you to the folks who hired me to do workshops and lectures and performances over the years, bring disability justice space onto campus, and kept me marginally employed. There are too many to name, but I want to say an especial thank you to Teal Van Dyck, Mateo Medina, Samantha Levens, Cascades, Eze Klarnet and Tash of the D Center, Eunjung Kim, Michael Gill, Tina Zavitsanos, Amalle Dublon, and Sylvie Rosenkalt.

Most of all, thank you to everyone who creates disability justice by doing the underappreciated disabled femme labor of listening (including via ASL and text and gesture and augmented communication), checking in, creating care teams and crisis teams, making soup and feeding people, helping lift heavy things, sharing cars and rides, fixing the ramp when it breaks, fundraising to buy accessible vans, sharing ramps, captioning videos, creating accessible venue lists, doing access audits, sniffing folks at the door, turning the lights down, creating ASL vlogs and fundraising for good interpretation, cocreating fragrance-free products for Black and brown hair and skin, hauling the air purifier and the accessible toilet seat to the show, making art and healing spaces, and passing on the last twenty dollars and handing over two Effexors. Thank you for being the crips who show up through vomit, level-9 pain days, nervous breakdowns, neurotypical and audist oppression, and inaccessible transit. Whenever anyone asks where they can find the disability justice movement, my answer is, it's here.

Lisa Factora-Borchers is the dream feminist of color editor I always needed and never found 'til now. After decades of struggling with racist and ableist editors where I spent most of my editing time fighting to stop them from writing all the brown, working-class, disabled language out of my work, it has been a miraculous gift to have an incredible Filipina feminist editor who skipped all that bullshit and just focused on making this book better. Thank you from the bottom of my heart for your deep brown Asian love and commitment to this work and for your years of devotion to amplifying feminist of color survivor voices. I am also grateful to Brian Lam, Cynara Geissler, and the entire team at Arsenal Pulp for the risks you take to champion QTBIPOC, disabled, femme, and survivor literary voices.

Throughout the thirteen years I have been publishing books, it has always been important to me for my books to feature beautiful pieces of art on the cover, created by QTBIPOC artists: thank you a million times to my friend TextaQueen and designer Oliver McPartlin for making a cover beautiful enough for this book that gives a visual language to queer brown disability that breaks away from the expected.

I wrote this book with images of and books by sick and disabled ancestors ringing my desk. I wrote this with their support and witness. Often when I got stuck, I would ask them what was needed. I call their names: Baba Ibrahim Farajajé , Audre Lorde, Frida Kahlo, Gloria Anzaldúa, Marsha P. Johnson, June Jordan, Taueret Davis, my great aunty Stasia Piepzna Smolon, Leslie Feinberg, Galvarino, Jerika Bolen, and Laura Hershey.

Finally, thank you to my beloved, Jesse Manuel Graves, for your love and kindness, Queen's femme snark, and brilliance. Every day with you is a miracle. Us finding each other and practicing love and care is our sick, disabled, and survivor ancestors' wildest dreams come true. And mine too.

"Crip Sex Moments and the Lust of Recognition: A Conversation with E.T. Russian" first appeared on the blog *Leaving Evidence*, May 25, 2010, https://leavingevidence.wordpress.com/2010/05/25/video-crip-sex-crip-lust-and-the-lust-of-recognition/.

"Cripping the Apocalypse: Some of My Wild Disability Justice Dreams" first appeared on *Truthout* as "To Survive the Trumpapocalypse, We Need Wild Disability Justice Dreams," May 20, 2018, https://truthout.org/articles/to-survive-the-trumpocalypse-we-need-wild-disability-justice-dreams/.

"For Badass Disability Justice, Working-Class and Poor-Led Models of Sustainable Hustling for Liberation" was published in *Organizing Upgrade,* Summer 2012.

"Fuck the 'Triumph of the Human Spirit': On Writing *Dirty River* as a Queer Disabled Femme-of-Color Memoir and the Joys of Saying Fuck You to Traditional Abuse Survivor Narratives" was published on www.thirdwomanpulse.com, September 17, 2015.

"Making Space Accessible Is an Act of Love for Our Communities" appeared in an earlier form on *Creating Collective Access*, June 2010, https://creatingcollectiveaccess.wordpress.com/.

"A Modest Proposal for a Fair Trade Emotional Labor Economy (Centered by Disabled, Femme of Color, Working-Class/Poor Genius)" first appeared in *Bitch*, Summer 2017.

"Not Over It, Not Fixed, and Living a Life Worth Living: Towards an Anti-Ableist Vision of Survivorhood" is forthcoming in *Whatever Gets You Through* (Vancouver: Greystone Books, 2019).

"Sick and Crazy Healer: A Not-So-Brief Personal History of the Healing Justice Movement" appeared in an earlier version as "A Not-So-Brief Personal History of the Healing Justice Movement, 2010–2016" in *MICE* magazine, no. 2, 2016.

"So Much Time Spent in Bed: A Letter to Gloria Anzaldúa on Chronic Illness, Coatlicue, and Creativity" originally appeared as a segment of "Sweet Dark Places," an essay cowritten by Qwo-Li Driskill and Aurora Levins Morales, in *El Mundo Zurdo 2* (San Francisco: Aunt Lute Books, 2012).

An earlier version of "Toronto Crip City: A Not-So-Brief, Incomplete Personal History of Some Moments in Time, 1997–2015" is forthcoming in *Marvellous Grounds: Queer of Colour Formations in Toronto* (Toronto: Between the Lines, 2018).

PREFACE

WRITING (WITH) A MOVEMENT FROM BED

When I moved to Oakland in 2007, I started writing from bed. I wrote in old sleep pants, lying on a heating pad, during the hours I spent in my big sick-and-disabled femme of color bed cave. I wasn't alone in this. I did so alongside many other sick and disabled writers making culture. Writing from bed is a time-honored disabled way of being an activist and cultural worker. It's one the mainstream doesn't often acknowledge but whose lineage stretches from Frida Kahlo painting in bed to Grace Lee Boggs writing in her wheelchair at age ninety-eight.

I had very good timing. I moved to Oakland just as disability justice was birthing itself as a movement. "Disability justice" is a term coined by the Black, brown, queer, and trans members of the original Disability Justice Collective, founded in 2005 by Patty Berne, Mia Mingus, Leroy Moore, Eli Clare, and Sebastian Margaret. Disabled queer and trans Black, Asian, and white activists and artists, they dreamed up a movement-building framework that would center the lives, needs, and organizing strategies of disabled queer and trans and/or Black and brown people marginalized from mainstream disability rights organizing's white-dominated, single-issue focus. Sins Invalid[1], the disability justice performance collective cocreated by Patty Berne and Leroy Moore, was based in Oakland and was shaking things up with its large-scale, beautifully produced performances about Black and brown queer disabled sex, bodies, and struggles, its use of culture as a weapon to reshape people's dreams, nightmares, and future visions of disabled Black and brown queer liberation. The

---

1   For more about Sins Invalid's vibrant history as a performance collective, see http://sinsinvalid.org/ or https://youtube.com/CripJustice.

writing of disabled queer Black and brown writers and activists like Mia Mingus, Stacey Milbern, Aurora Levins Morales, and Billie Rain was shaking things up online and in print, their pieces being passed from hand to hand in communities I was part of. I was reading them over and over again, silently in my room, my brain breaking open. I had never seen disabled queer and trans Black, Indigenous, and people of color (QTBIPOC) writers talking about the nitty-gritty facts of our lives out loud before, without apology. It felt like queer crip of color writers were creating space for sick and disabled queer and trans people of color to name ourselves as disabled, our kind of disabled, for the first time, and talk about the shit we'd only whispered before. We were finding ourselves, and each other, and making sick and disabled QTBIPOC space that held our desires and our stories. It felt like some non-disabled queers and activists were paying attention, being forced to deal with ableism, and with us, whether or not they were thrilled about it.

As disability justice was giving birth to itself as a movement, I got to be part of it as a cultural worker, often working from bed. As I was able to perform with Sins Invalid and experienced its exquisitely high level of access for disabled artists, that experience refused to stay in one little corner of my life—I wanted all the QTBIPOC cultural spaces I took part in to be that accessible, that whole. I wrote pieces about cross-disability access that were tools I and other disabled BIPOC queers and allies used to help create the first Creating Collective Access network[2], an experiment in access made by and for QTBIPOC disabled people at the 2010 Allied Media Conference (AMC) and US Social Forum (USSF) that broke away from traditional formats of "access as service begrudgingly offered to disabled people

---

2   For more information about the CCA, check out https://creatingcollectiveaccess .wordpress.com/. I talk in more detail about the CCA in "Care Webs: Experiments in Creating Collective Access" (see p. 32).

by non-disabled people who feel grumpy about it" to "access as a collective joy and offering we can give to each other." Finding other disabled QTBIPOC creators and building with them prompted me to write about what it meant to create performing arts spaces where access was a central part of the performance, not an afterthought. As queers and femmes in my communities, particularly queer femmes of color and multiply marginalized femmes, continued to kill themselves, I wrote about suicidality as an ever-present reality in our communities. As I finally finished my first memoir after ten years of work, I wrote about what it takes to write femme of color disabled trauma stories and how survivorhood is part of disability justice.

I wrote these pieces not out of a desire for fame or cultural capital but to be useful. Culture makes culture. When there's no space to talk about disability in art—when people at the poetry slam respond to your crip poem with "How touching" and give you sad face, or just look confused—disabled artists of color won't make disabled art. When there are few QTBIPOC arts spaces, QTBIPOC tend to think art isn't a viable career option. Disability justice allowed me to understand that me writing from my sickbed wasn't me being weak or uncool or not a real writer but a time-honored crip creative practice. And that understanding allowed me to finally write from a disabled space, for and about sick and disabled people, including myself, without feeling like I was writing about boring, private things that no one would understand.

This is a big deal. Because, while I got sick with fibromyalgia and chronic fatigue immune deficiency syndrome (CFIDS)[3] in 1997, and have been a neurodivergent survivor of violence with complex PTSD all my life, I didn't write or publish anything about disability until *Bodymap*, my third book of poetry, came out in 2015. It was almost twenty years

---

3   The term most commonly used now, like on official websites and the like, is "Chronic Fatigue Immune Dysfunction," but I learned it as "chronic fatigue immune deficiency syndrome," and that's what I've been using for twenty-plus years, so I think we'll stick with it.

since I'd first become chronically ill and a decade into my publishing books. Before I had the great good fortune to run into Sins Invalid and other queer people of color talking and writing about disability, I, like many other QTBIPOC I knew, thought of disability as something that you weren't allowed to talk or write about in QTBIPOC culture. Nowhere in the QTBIPOC politicized spoken word communities I was part of (or wanted to be cool enough to be part of) in the early 2000s do I remember anyone ever doing poetry about disability or thinking about access at all. (Do you remember any poems about disability justice making it onto *Def Poetry Jam*? I don't.) And that state of affairs continued into my adult life in the able-bodied QTBIPOC artist community. It's not like anyone came right out and said they hated disabled people. But disability was depressing or embarrassing to write about, or just something that "most people wouldn't be able to relate to as a subject." There was a huge echoing silence in POC and/or queer activist communities. I had a few friends who whispered to each other about our chronic illnesses—but the most we could say was "It sucks, right?" We had no idea we could be part of a community, a history, a movement.

But in the past decade, disability justice culture has bloomed, through the hard work of disabled people who are also queer feminists of color, and it's not like that anymore—at least, not all of the time. It's not that ableist disregard for crip lives, both in the mainstream and inside our movements and communities, doesn't still exist. But I no longer worry that every single person I encounter at an event will be awkward or pity me or just not get it. I do not feel like I am the only person I know who is talking about disability justice. I no longer feel like one of a tiny handful of people talking about access or worry that if I produce a crip show of course no one will come to it. I think more people know that not all disabled people are white. When I first started offering sick and disabled writing workshops for queer and trans people of color around 2010, sometimes no one would come out, or just a few people, or the idea would be shot down because the organizers were sure no one would come. But when I went on tour with *Bodymap* in 2015 and read explicitly disability-focused work, almost all of my gigs were standing and sitting room only. When I did a writing workshop by and for sick and disabled people of color at the 2015 Queer Students of Color Conference, the room was spilling over with queer people of color who wanted to talk and write about everything from pesticide exposures they had received doing farm work to intergenerational trauma. Disabled Black and brown queer voices are no longer uncommon on popular feminist and queer blogs like *The Body Is Not an Apology, Everyday Feminism, GUTS,* and *Autostraddle,* and I see articles including and thinking about ableism instead of forgetting about it. The Disability Visibility Project, Wear Your Voice, the Spoonie Collective, the Deaf Poets Society, Autistic Hoya, Krip-Hop Nation, and many other sites by and for intersectional disabled people are live. Everywhere people are talking about care work, emotional labor, femme emotional labor, access, and crip skills and science.

None of this happened because the able-bodied people decided to be nice to the cripples. It happened because disabled queer and trans people of color started organizing, often with femme disabled Black and brown queer people in the lead. Much of that work has been done through writing, storytelling, and art as activism. Much of our coming together has been through zines, online disabled QT/POC communities, Tumblr and blog and social media posts, or through three people getting together at a kitchen table or a group Skype call to start to hesitantly talk about our lives, organize a meal train, share pills and tips, or post the thoughts about activism and survival we have at two in the morning. It is underdocumented, private work—work often seen as not "real activism." But it is the realest activism there is. This is how disability justice art and activism change the world and save lives.

In writing this book, I wanted to capture some of this history as it is being made and dreamed.

CONCRETE TOOLS, LIBERATION POLITICS, AND POETRY
THIS IS DISABILITY JUSTICE

I'd like to offer a quick definition and history of what we mean when we say the words "disability justice." This is important for so many reasons but especially because our work and terminology are in danger, now and always, of having the fact that they were invented by Black, Indigenous, and people of color erased and their politics watered down. There is a specific danger in that happening with disability justice, as disabled Black and brown creators face a specific invisibilization and erasure of our political and cultural work. I want to both give the Black and brown people and femmes who invented the term credit and be clear about what DJ means and what it doesn't.

In the words of Sins Invalid cofounder and executive director Patty Berne,

> While a concrete and radical move forward toward justice for disabled people, the Disability Rights Movement simultaneously invisibilized the lives of peoples who lived at intersecting junctures of oppression—disabled people of color, immigrants with disabilities, queers with disabilities, trans and gender non-conforming people with disabilities, people with disabilities who are houseless, people with disabilities who are incarcerated, people with disabilities who have had their ancestral lands stolen, amongst others ... Disability Justice activists, organizers, and cultural workers understand that able-bodied supremacy has been formed in relation to other systems of domination and exploitation. The histories of white supremacy and ableism

are inextricably entwined, both forged in the crucible of colonial conquest and capitalist domination. One cannot look at the history of US slavery, the stealing of indigenous lands, and US imperialism without seeing the way that white supremacy leverages ableism to create a subjugated 'other' that is deemed less worthy/abled/smart/capable ... We cannot comprehend ableism without grasping its interrelations with heteropatriarchy, white supremacy, colonialism and capitalism. Each system benefits from extracting profits and status from the subjugated 'other.' 500+ years of violence against black and brown communities includes 500+ years of bodies and minds deemed 'dangerous' by being non-normative.

A Disability Justice framework understands that all bodies are unique and essential, that all bodies have strengths and needs that must be met. We know that we are powerful not despite the complexities of our bodies, but because of them ... Disability Justice holds a vision born out of collective struggle, drawing upon the legacies of cultural and spiritual resistance within a thousand underground paths, igniting small persistent fires of rebellion in everyday life. Disabled people of the global majority—black and brown people—share common ground confronting and subverting colonial powers in our struggle for life and justice. There has always been resistance to all forms of oppression, as we know through our bones that there have simultaneously been disabled people visioning a world where we flourish, that values and celebrates us in all our myriad beauty.[4]

---

4   Patty Berne, "Skin, Tooth, and Bone—The Basis of Our Movement Is People: A Disability Justice Primer," *Reproductive Health Matters* 25, no. 50 (May 2017): 149–50.

To me, disability justice means a political movement and many interlocking communities where disability is not defined in white terms, or male terms, or straight terms. Disability justice is to the disability rights movement what the environmental justice movement is to the mainstream environmental movement. Disability justice centers sick and disabled people of color, queer and trans disabled folks of color, and everyone who is marginalized in mainstream disability organizing.

More than that, disability justice asserts that ableism helps make racism, christian supremacy, sexism, and queer- and transphobia possible, and that all those systems of oppression are locked up tight. It insists that we organize from our sick, disabled, "brokenbeautiful" (as Alexis Pauline Gumbs[5] puts it) bodies' wisdom, need, and desire. It means looking at how Indigenous and Black and brown traditions value sick and disabled folks (not as magical cripples but as people of difference whose bodyspirits have valuable smarts), at how in BIPOC communities being sick or disabled can just be "life," and also at how sick and disabled BIPOC are criminalized. It means asserting a vision of liberation in which destroying ableism is part of social justice. It means the hotness, smarts, and value of our sick and disabled bodies. It means we are not left behind; we are beloved, kindred, needed.

When we do disability justice work, it becomes impossible to look at disability and not examine how colonialism created it. It becomes a priority to look at Indigenous ways of perceiving and understanding disability, for example. It becomes a space where we see that disability is all up in Black and brown/queer and trans communities—from Henrietta Lacks to Harriet Tubman, from the Black Panther Party's active support for disabled organizers' two-month occupation of the Department of Vocational Rehabilitation to force the passage of

---

5   Alexis Pauline Gumbs, brokenbeautiful press, https://brokenbeautiful.wordpress.com, accessed May 28, 2018.

Section 504, the law mandating disabled access to public spaces and transportation to the chronic illness and disability stories of second-wave queer feminists of color like Sylvia Rivera, June Jordan, Gloria Anzaldúa, Audre Lorde, Marsha P. Johnson, and Barbara Cameron, whose lives are marked by bodily difference, trauma-surviving brilliance, and chronic illness but who mostly never used the term "disabled" to refer to themselves. Many of us rely on state funding and services to survive and fight for things like the Affordable Care Act (ACA) and the Americans with Disabilities Act (ADA) to remain protected and expanded. But our focus is less on civil rights legislation as the only solution to ableism and more on a vision of liberation that understands that the state was built on racist, colonialist ableism and will not save us, because it was created to kill us. A movement where, in the words of Sins Invalid, "we move together, with no body left behind."

To me, one quality of disability justice culture is that it is simultaneously beautiful and practical. Poetry and dance are as valuable as a blog post about access hacks—because they're equally important and interdependent. This book is an example of that both/and. In this mosaic, you will find pieces of personal testimony and poetry, meditations on Gloria Anzaldúa and Prince as disabled queer Black and brown figures, grassroots intellectual examinations of accessible performance spaces as prefigurative politics—and tips for how to tour as a chronically ill artist and notes on where to get accessible fragrance-free POC hair products.

That is not usual, and that is on purpose. Like disability justice itself as a framework and culture, this book is a mix of very concrete tools and personal essays. I hesitated a bit to include the former. Serious cultural work isn't supposed to include lists of fragrance-free curly hair products or instructions about how to tour while sick and hurt less, right? But—*fuck that*. The making of disability justice lives in the realm of thinking and talking and knowledge making, in art and sky. But it also lives in how to rent an accessible porta potty for an accessible-except-the-bathroom event space, how to mix coconut oil and aloe to make a fragrance-free hair lotion that works for curly and kinky BIPOC hair, how to learn to care for each other when everyone is sick, tired, crazy, and brilliant. And neither is possible without the other.

CARE WORK IN THE APOCALYPSE

When I began working on this book in July 2016—right after I quit the job at a giant corporate university that I had hoped would be an accessible way of making a living but ended up giving me pneumonia for three months—I thought I'd just slap together a collection of all the pieces of writing I'd done over the past decade: essays about curating QTBIPOC performance art, the *Femme Shark Manifesto*. But as I edited this book over the summer of 2017, I realized that the pieces that were the most prominent were all ones that I'd written about disability justice and care labor in many forms.

The theme of care work, as a place where disability justice and queer femme emotional labor intersect, came to me. "Nothing about us without us" is a disability rights slogan that was created by South African disability rights groups in the 1980s. A more recent disability justice slogan I have heard, that I first saw on an image Sins Invalid created in protest of the killing intersections of racism and ableism in the Israeli bombardment of Gaza in the summer of 2014, is "To exist is to resist." This phrase speaks to the ways in which the everyday struggles to live and survive by sick and disabled QTBIPOC are "real" activism—when you are lying in bed trying to breathe or talking someone through a panic attack or fighting Medicaid or the queer club to let you in, that is resistance. And in this political moment, where Trump is attempting to kill sick and disabled people by ending Medicaid, the Affordable Care Act, and the ADA, and where the things that do save us—emergent airport demonstrations against Trump's Islamophobic and racist travel and immigration bans, care webs where we raise money for medical and housing surpluses—are so clearly not the state, this book feels timely.

I also wrote this book with a lot of anxiety. I was very conscious during the process of compiling and editing this book that it would be the first on disability justice by a queer writer of color that was not self- or micropress-published. This is huge, and telling: that the racism and ableism of the publishing industry mean there are barely any popular books out there on disability, and the vast majority of them are written by white, disabled people. Like every other disabled writer I know, I have been asked if I think "readers will really know what ableism is." I have had pieces about disability politics be read with incomprehension by editors who said, "Don't you want to say more about your illness?" and were confused that I am not telling the only disabled story they can comprehend—a simple, tragic yet uplifting tale where I talk about my "illness" and how I have "overcome" it—but a story of collective struggle, community building, love and luck and skills. Like every disabled Black and brown writer I know, I have fought to get anyone to give a shit or not just throw up their hands at how way too complicated my story is—can't I just focus on my brownness or ableism?

Because I am a cultural worker who is one disabled femme of color writer in a collective movement of many, I was clear about what I did and did not want this book to be. For the past year, I have thought a lot about what I wanted to do to intervene in the very likely reality that, as I am a light-skinned, non-Black, ambulatory, often verbally communicative person, mainstream media would want to cast me as "the face of disability justice" and thrust into the spotlight as the one "expert" on this wacky new movement—erasing all of my comrades and fellow artists, thinkers, and organizers, particularly those who face certain kinds of ableism that are more overt and killing than some that I face. This fear didn't come from nowhere: I had one offer to publish this book that meant very well in talking about how "the time had come for a big book on disability justice" but then admitted that in mainstream publishing, unless you're willing to pitch yourself as "the expert," essay books don't sell.

I am and want to be very clear: I am one writer and performer in a sea of sick and disabled QT/BIPOC people who are doing work in many ways all the time—as writers and activists, and as everyday folks who are keeping themselves and other people alive. I do not want this to be "the" book on disability justice. This book is one in a garden of books that I invoke to become more abundant. Please check out the books, authors, websites, and zines in the Further Reading and Resources section for a complete view of what this world is.

But for now, please come into this one. And write your own.

10 PRINCIPLES OF DISABILITY JUSTICE

by Patty Berne, edited by Aurora Levins Morales and David Langstaff, on behalf of Sins Invalid

From my vantage point within Sins Invalid, where we incubate both the framework and practice of Disability Justice, this burgeoning framework has ten (10) principles, each offering new opportunities for movement builders:

1. INTERSECTIONALITY. We know that each person has multiple identities, and that each identity can be a site of privilege or oppression. The mechanical workings of oppression and how they output shift depending upon the characteristics of any given institutional or interpersonal interaction; the very understanding of disability experience itself is being shaped by race, gender, class, gender expression, historical moment, relationship to colonization, and more.

2. LEADERSHIP OF THOSE MOST IMPACTED. We know ableism exists in the context of other historical systemic oppressions. We know to truly have liberation we must be led by those who know the most about these systems and how they work.

3. ANTI-CAPITALIST POLITIC. We are anti-capitalist, as the very nature of our mind/bodies often resists conforming to a capitalist "normative" level of production. We don't believe human worth is dependent on what and how much a person can produce. We critique a concept of "labor" as defined by able-bodied supremacy, white supremacy, and gender normativity. We understand capitalism to be a system that promotes private wealth accumulation for some at the expense of others.

4. CROSS-MOVEMENT SOLIDARITY. Necessarily cross movement, Disability Justice shifts how social justice movements understand disability and contextualize ableism, lending itself towards a united front politic.

5. RECOGNIZING WHOLENESS. We value our people as they are, for who they are, and understand that people have inherent worth outside of capitalist notions of productivity. Each person is full of history and life experience. Each person has an internal experience composed of their own thoughts, sensations, emotions, sexual fantasies, perceptions, and idiosyncrasies. Disabled people are whole people.

6. SUSTAINABILITY. We pace ourselves, individually and collectively, to be sustained long term. We value the teachings of our lives and bodies. We understand that our embodied experience is a critical guide and reference pointing us toward justice and liberation.

7. COMMITMENT TO CROSS-DISABILITY SOLIDARITY. We value and honor the insights and participation of all of our community members.

We are committed to breaking down ableist/patriarchal/racist/classed isolation between people with physical impairments, people who identify as "sick" or are chronically ill, "psych" survivors and those who identify as "crazy," neurodiverse people, people with cognitive impairments, and people who are of a sensory minority, as we understand that isolation ultimately undermines collective liberation.

8. INTERDEPENDENCE. Before the massive colonial project of Western European expansion, we understood the nature of interdependence within our communities. We see the liberation of all living systems and the land as integral to the liberation of our own communities, as we all share one planet. We attempt to meet each other's needs as we build towards liberation, without always reaching for state solutions that inevitably then extend its control further over our lives.

9. COLLECTIVE ACCESS. As brown/black and queer crips, we bring flexibility and creative nuance to engage with each other. We create and explore new ways of doing things that go beyond able-bodied/minded normativity. Access needs aren't shameful—we all have various capacities which function differently in various environments. Access needs can be articulated within a community and met privately or through a collective, depending upon an individual's needs, desires, and the capacity of the group. We can share responsibility for our access needs, we can ask that our needs be met without compromising our integrity, we can balance autonomy while being in community, we can be unafraid of our vulnerabilities knowing our strengths are respected.

10. COLLECTIVE LIBERATION. How do we move together as people with mixed abilities, multiracial, multi-gendered, mixed class, across the orientation spectrum—where no body/mind is left behind?

This is Disability Justice, an honoring of the long-standing legacies of resilience and resistance which are the inheritance of all of us whose bodies or minds will not conform. Disability Justice is not yet a broad-based popular movement. Disability Justice is a vision and practice of a *yet-to-be*, a map that we create with our ancestors and our great-grandchildren onward, in the width and depth of our multiplicities and histories, a movement towards a world in which every body and mind is known as beautiful.

PART
I

CARE WEBS

EXPERIMENTS IN CREATING COLLECTIVE ACCESS

Do you have the car today? Hayati, I'm at the bus stop, I hurt so bad, can you pick me up? Hey, can I borrow twenty dollars? Can you go buy groceries for me when you're out and drop them off? Here's a list. Do you want to go to community acupuncture together? Hey, B. needs more care shifters, can you repost this Facebook note? Can we share the access van ride over to the city? If you come, you can say you're my personal care attendant and you won't have to pay. Do you have anemone tincture[6] you could bring over? I'm flaring. Holding me would be good too. If I take your manual wheelchair and load it up with takeout, we'll all have food. Can you go with me to the clinic and take notes while I talk to my doctor? Can I use your address for the Easy Does It pickup?[7] I'm just over the border into Oakland. Let's pass the hat so we can afford ASL for the event. Do you have the interpreter list? Here's the list of accessible event spaces we made on Google docs. Can you be part of my mad map[8] crisis fam? Wanna Skype if you can't get out, even if we live in the same city? Wanna go with me to the food stamp office? Can you pick up an eighth for me when you go to the dispensary?

---

6   Anemone is an herb that can be used for anxiety and panic attacks.

7   Easy Does It is a wheelchair accessible van service that operates in Berkeley, California.

8   A "mad map" is a term invented by the Icarus Project, a care plan used to describe what madness looks like for a person and what care they do or do not want. For more information, see https://theicarusproject.net/.

What does it mean to shift our ideas of access and care (whether it's disability, childcare, economic access, or many more) from an individual chore, an unfortunate cost of having an unfortunate body, to a collective responsibility that's maybe even deeply joyful?

What does it mean for our movements? Our communities/fam? Ourselves and our own lived experience of disability and chronic illness?

What does it mean to wrestle with these ideas of softness and strength, vulnerability, pride, asking for help, and not—all of which are so deeply raced and classed and gendered?

If collective access is revolutionary love without charity, how do we learn to love each other? How do we learn to do this love work of collective care that lifts us instead of abandons us, that grapples with all the deep ways in which care is complicated?

This is an essay about care—about the ways sick and disabled people attempt to get the care and support we need, on our own terms, with autonomy and dignity. It's specifically an essay about some experiments that have taken place over the past decade by sick and disabled predominantly Black and brown queer people to create networks of care by and for us. It's about our attempts to get what we need to love and live, interdependently, in the world and in our homes, without primarily relying on the state or, often, our biological families—the two sources disabled and sick people have most often been forced to rely on for care, sometimes, well, often, with abuse and lack of control. This is about some of the ways we are attempting to dream ways to access care deeply, in a way where we are in control, joyful, building community, loved, giving, and receiving, that doesn't burn anyone out or abuse or underpay anyone in the process. This is for us and by us, and it is also for everyone who thinks of themselves as able-bodied and normatively minded, who may not be, who will not always be, who the ghost of the need for care still dances with as deepest fate-worse-than-death fear, as what you want the most but can't even let yourself speak.

It is an essay full of sick and disabled QTBIPOC stories that are well known in certain activist disabled QTBIPOC circles but at risk of disappearing or not being passed down, as the mediums where we find each other become less accessible/safe (Facebook in the age of Trump) or fade away (Web 2.0). And I am also thinking of care webs that have existed through time, that I know of through queer legend and myth, that do not often get counted as disabled stories and may not have thought of themselves as disabled care stories but still shared access tools, meds, and care—STAR House, the house started by Black and brown trans femme sex worker revolutionaries Marsha P. Johnson and Sylvia Rivera, with the rent paid by hustling and street sex work, as a safe space for trans people of color and street trans people to be free, be with each other, and share hormones and other supplies for healing and gender affirmation; the AIDS activist prisoner networks in the 1980s and '90s that shared safer sex supplies and AIDS drugs and fought for prisoners to receive medical care; the mad movement's underground safe houses and sharing of both pills and alternative treatments, as well as ways of coming off meds safely; the underground, often criminalized, harm-reduction networks like the New England Drug Users Union today where people share naloxone and fentanyl testing strips in their living rooms with folks who use opioids. We have found each other and offered healing and access to each other before and will again.

It is an essay full of questions. About what allows us to access care, as sick and disabled people who have been taught that our care needs are a pain in the ass and a burden—to the economy, the state, our families, the person we have to share the bus stop with so we need to take up as small a space as possible. It is an essay rooted in the stories I know, live, and witness, as a working-class, disabled femme of color—of all the ways our people have saved and continue to save each other against huge odds. It is an essay about the miracles that sick and disabled communities of color make for each other, and it's also about the contradictions and the cracks. Some of the questions are about what stops us from being able to ask for care when we come from Black and brown communities, for example, who have always been the ones forced to care for others for little or no money. Or about what happens when sick and disabled people are the only ones who do not forget about each other, but we all are extremely, extremely tired. I wrote this essay because I passionately believe in the power of our stories—of the revolution work we do when we cook a meal for each other, listen without judgment, share meds, hang out with each other during a psychotic break, or lift each other onto a toilet or a scooter.

I wrote this essay because I passionately believe in recording sick and disabled QTBIPOC stories, and because I believe the stories I have witnessed and participated in over the past decade of building ways of creating care are both a core part of disability justice work and the work of making the next world, the world we want, the post-Trump, post-fascist, postapocalyptic world. I wrote this because I believe we stand at the crossroads, between both the gifts and the unexpected, inevitable collapses of our work, and we have the opportunity to dream and keep dreaming ways to build emergent, resilient care webs. I believe that our work in creating the new world depends on it—because all of us will become disabled and sick, because state systems are failing, yet "community" is not a magic unicorn, a one-stop shop that always helps us do the laundry and be held in need. I believe that the only way we will do this is by being fucking real, by not papering over the places where our rhetoric falls flat, where we ran out of steam, or where this shit is genuinely fucking hard.

I wrote this for my mother, a working-class survivor of severe childhood sexual and physical abuse, a disabled Irish and Roma woman living with post-polio syndrome and no medical care, and then cancer spawned by environmental racism, as well as DID and complex PTSD, who was rarely if ever able to access any form of care or support for her disabilities, who both neglected me medically and shielded me from institutionalization as a young disabled and neurodivergent person, who did the absolute best and most common thing she could do as a working-class survivor who trusted no system and few people. I wrote this for my younger self, a newly incredibly sick, isolated twenty-two-year-old, who made up ways to care for my disabilities in isolation from disability community, from books, prayers, guessing, and dreams. I wrote this for everyone who has been denied SSI, SSDI, ODSP, or whatever they call state disability money where you live, or "official" disability accommodations for the first or fourth time, who can't get that "medical proof" of our sickness or disability and who thus can't get anything the state begrudgingly offers us—that discounted transit, Access-A-Ride, state or federal disability benefits, welfare, accommodations at school or work. This is for those of us who are closeting our disability to keep everything from health insurance and jobs to social acceptance and capital—all of which we need to survive.

This is for those of us who cannot closet our disability, Madness, Deafness, and illness—whose witnessable disability is just a fact of life that becomes a bullet target for violence, for attempts by police, doctors, and families to murder us and lock us up. This is for all of us evading that capture and control, that being disposed of—who still have need. This is for everyone Black and brown who freeze, who feel we could never, ever think about asking someone to do our dishes or clean our toilet or help us dress, because that is the work we or our families have done for little or no money during enslavement, colonial invasion, immigration, and racist poverty—and this is for those of us who have both cleaned toilets and wiped asses for little or no pay and respect and who too need and deserve care with respect and dignity. This is for all of us, especially Black, Indigenous, and brown femme people, who have kept our communities alive after being both abandoned and policed by the state, and in the face of medical experimentation and denial of health insurance.

This is for all the friends I know who have needed care but also needed to evade Children's Aid and foster care. This is for everyone who desperately needs care but will never let a care worker in their house for fear they or their children will be taken away by the state. This is for everyone who has had to run away from accepting care because care meant control—by family members or partners or workers or strangers. This is for every group of stressed-out QTBIPOC friends who are the only three disabled people you know, who are doing all the care for each other until it trails away into frustration, stress, yelling, and breakdowns. This is for those of us who have been forgotten and left behind by our communities, who have and have not survived that abandonment and isolation. This is for everyone trying to keep themselves or their friend out of the psych ward, who sometimes want more than anything for some actual professional who wouldn't be messed up and who would actually help. This is for all the times I've relaxed into the miracle of being cared for well, that changed my understanding of what was possible, and every time I've succeeded and failed at caring well. This is for the road we make by moving forward, the dream future of autonomous care we deserve.

HOW PEOPLE GET CARE (AND DON'T) AND WHAT CARE MEANS

I'm not an academically trained disability scholar, and I'm not going to pretend that this next section fits (white-dominated) disability studies academic standards. The history of disabled people accessing or being denied care and the ways our needs have been policed and profited off of is vast, and there is no way I can do it justice in one essay—but I wanted to offer a very brief history of how care has and has not been offered to us in North America pre- and post-colonialism. (I am also aware of how so much writing about disability is limited to a white-dominated disability studies field and language, and how inaccessible that is to the vast majority of sick and disabled people who could potentially use it—so there are pros and cons to both approaches.) But here goes: There have been a million ways sick and disabled people have accessed the care we need over the centuries, and I don't have time to go over them. A light once-over will say that in many precolonial contact communities, there existed ways of being disabled that did not mean stigma, shame, exile, or death. Disabled Cherokee scholar Qwo-Li Driskill has remarked that in precontact Cherokee, there are many words for people with different kinds of bodies, illnesses, and what would be seen as impairments; none of those words are negative or view those sick or disabled people as defective or not as good as normatively bodied people.[9]

With the arrival of white settler colonialism, things changed, and not in a good way. For many sick and disabled Black, Indigenous, and brown people under transatlantic enslavement, colonial invasion, and forced labor, there was no such thing as state-funded care. Instead, if we were too sick or disabled to work, we were often killed, sold, or left to die, because we were not making factory or plantation owners money. Sick, disabled, Mad, Deaf, and neurodivergent people's care and treatment varied according to our race, class, gender, and location, but for the most part, at best, we were able to evade capture and find ways of caring for ourselves or being cared for by our families, nations, or communities—from our Black and brown communities to disabled communities. At worst, a combination of legal and societal ableism plus racism and colonialism meant that we were locked up in institutions or hospitals, "for our own good." The Ugly Laws, on the books in

---

9   Qwo-Li Driskill, personal conversation with the author, August 2011.

the United States from the mid-1700s to the 1970s, stated that many disabled people were "too ugly" to be in public and legally prevented disabled people from being able to take up space in public. The Ugly Laws were interwoven with a mass creation in the 1800s and onward of hospitals, "homes," "sanitoriums," and "charitable institutions" where it was the norm for disabled, sick, mad, and Deaf people to be sequestered from able-bodied "normal society."[10]

These institutions overlapped with other prison/carceral systems, like residential schools, where Indigenous children were stolen, abused, and stripped of their language and culture, and prisons where Black, brown, poor, criminalized, trans, queer, and sex working people were locked up for profit. People's fear of accessing care didn't come out of nowhere. It came out of generations and centuries where needed care meant being locked up, losing your human and civil rights, and being subject to abuse. The specter of "the home" and lockup still haunts everyone when we consider asking for or needing care.

One of the first and most passionate demands of the disability rights and mental patients liberation movements of the 1960s and '70s was for independent living and deinstitutionalization. It's an often-told crip story—how the disability rights movement started with the Rolling Quads, the white, polio-surviving, physically disabled men who got radicalized while attending UC Berkeley by both witnessing Black and brown power and free speech movements and being sequestered in each other's company because they were only allowed to live in the campus infirmary. How after graduation, they started the first independent living centers and pushed for Medicare and Medicaid to

---

10   For more about this huge disabled history, see Eli Clare, *Brilliant Imperfection: Grappling with Cure* (Durham, NA: Duke University Press, 2017); Susan M. Schweik, *The Ugly Laws: Disability in Public* (New York: New York University Press, 2010); Sunaura Taylor, "After the Ugly Laws," *The Baffler*, February 28, 2017, https://thebaffler.com/blog/after-the-ugly-laws-taylor, and "I Want to Help the Handicapped ... According to the Charity Model of Disability," www.ju90.co.uk/help/eng/help1.

pay for state-funded personal care attendants to allow them to live in their own apartments and get help with dressing, using the bathroom, and transferring from bed to chair.

Yet some/many of us live in the "cliffhangers," as Patty Berne puts it, of the disability rights movement—the spaces where a white-dominated, single-issue, civil rights approach that depends on the ability to use lawsuits to achieve disability liberation leaves many of us behind. Some of us are disabled folks who are able to access care attendants to help us live that are paid for by the state, Department of Health, or Social Services. Some of us are disabled people whose disability the state never approves of—so it's not "real." Some of us fear that letting anyone in to care for us will mean we are declared incompetent and lose our civil rights, so we guard the houses where we can be sick. Some of us know that accepting care means accepting queerphobia, transphobia, fatphobia or sexphobia from our care attendants. Some of us are in the in-between of needing some care but not fitting into the state model of either Total and Permanent Disability or fit and ready to work—so we can't access the services that are there. Many of us are familiar with being genuinely sick as hell and needing some help but failing the official crip exams because we can still cook, shop, and work, only slowly and when there is no other choice. Some of us are not citizens. Some of us make twenty bucks too much. Some of us will lose our right to marry if we go on state disability, or our access to work or housing. Some of us belong to Nations that will not accept state money. Some of us—always, and especially post-Trump, with the rise of fascism calling for the end of Medicaid, the ACA, and the ADA in the US, and socialized medicine and human rights legislation throughout the world—are continuously worrying about what happens when our precarious right to state-funded care goes away, and what our survival strategies will be then.

MOVING PAST NIGHTMARE TOWARDS STRATEGIES FOR THE FUTURE OF COLLECTIVE ACCESS

In the face of systems that want us dead, sick and disabled people have been finding ways to care for ourselves and each other for a long time. As Vancouver's *Radical Access Mapping Project*[11] says, "Able-bodied people: if you don't know how to do access, ask disabled people. We've been doing it for a long time, usually on no money, and we're really good at it." Sometimes we call them care webs or collectives, sometimes we call them "my friend that helps me out sometimes," sometimes we don't call them anything at all—care webs are just life, just what you do.

The care webs I write about here break from the model of paid attendant care as the only way to access disability support. Resisting the model of charity and gratitude, they are controlled by the needs and desires of the disabled people running them. Some of them rely on a mix of abled and disabled people to help; some of them are experiments in "crip-made access"—access made by and for disabled people only, turning on its head the model that disabled people can only passively receive care, not give it or determine what kind of care we want. Whether they are disabled only or involve disabled and non-disabled folks, they still work from a model of *solidarity not charity*—of showing up for each other in mutual aid and respect.

I first learned of the term "mutual aid" as an anarchist teenager, in books like Ursula Le Guin's *The Dispossessed* and in a lot of zines that quoted white guy theorists like Kropotkin. All of these writers, and many other anarchist and antiauthoritarian writers, use the term to mean a voluntary reciprocal exchange of resources and services for mutual benefit. Mutual aid, as opposed to charity, does not connote moral superiority of the giver over the receiver. White people didn't invent the concept of mutual aid—many precolonial (and after) Black,

---

11   *Radical Access Mapping Project*, https://radicalaccessiblecommunities.wordpress.com.

Indigenous, and brown communities have complex webs of exchanges of care. However, given the presence of white anarchism as one of the biggest places that talk about ideas of mutual aid, it doesn't surprise me that one of the first examples of collective care I encountered was dreamed up by a white Southern disabled queer femme anarchist whose politics brought together disability and mutual aid.

THE PREQUEL: LOREE ERICKSON'S CARE COLLECTIVE

Hello Lovely People ...

For those of you who don't know me I am Loree Erickson, a queer femmegimp porn star academic who now lives in Toronto, ON but grew up in Leesburg, VA and lived in Richmond for 8 years. My work tends to focus on the inter-sections of radical queer, disability and sex/uality bringing together personal experience, creativity (through video and photography), and theory to explore issues of explicit sexual representation, embodiment, and desirability. As well I theorize around personal assistance/care relationships and create alternative support structures. I also love sun, sparkly things, and social justice. I am coming to DC to present at a day long seminar for and by young women with disabilities at American University. Then, of course I have to come to RVA and see my people (as well as eat biscuits and gravy at 821 Cafe).

I arrive in DC Friday, around 1ish and am around until Monday morning. Then I am heading to Richmond till Wednesday eve. I am traveling with a friend who can help out with some of my care, but I am in need of friendly recruits to help as well. Plus it's an awesome opportunity to meet fabulous and friendly people/see friends I have seen in too long!

How you can help:

I use a wheelchair and I am looking to recruit folks to help with my personal care needs (fancy words for getting into/out of bed and going to the bathroom). No experience needed (I am really good at talking folks through it plus what I need help with is pretty straight forward) and ya only have to be sorta buff. I [weigh] around 130lbs, but it is not as bad as it seems. If you're worried about lifting I might be able to buddy you up or maybe you can buddy yourself up with a friend. Two people makes it way easier and yay for safety! :-) It doesn't take that long (around a 1 hour—usually less—to pee and a bit more to get into/outta bed. I usually pee at 12ish, 5ish and then when I get into bed and wake up. If you don't have a lot of time, even one shift would be so extremely helpful.

If you are interested let me know or if you know anyone else who might be interested, please send this their way (I appreciate people of all genders helping me). I need to know as soon as possible so that I know how stressed out to be. Plus we are coming soo soon! :) Also if you can send me your availability that would be amazing.

Help with any part of this would be awesome and forwarding it to other nice people is also very much appreciated. Thanks soo much ...

Can't wait to see/meet you and your friends!!!

Loree

Interviewer: "Your model of collective care includes disability as part of our social understanding of mutual care. What you are doing is helping to shift our collective social understanding of care. It's profoundly political."

Loree Erickson: [Nods her head] "Yeah, it really is. It's too bad that taking care of each other has to be radical."[12]

Encountering Loree Erickson's artwork, and then learning about and witnessing her care collective, changed my life. Her artwork and disabled community organizing were some of the first places where I saw a femme disabled person talk about disability, femmeness, and desirability, or the concept of interdependence, or collective care as a thing that could exist in the world. Her queer femme anarchist disabled white Southern art, organizing, and self were everyday parts of my political reality in Toronto in the mid-2000s and had a huge impact on the city's activist communities. For many people in Toronto and beyond, her care collective has been both a groundbreaking model for alternative dreams of care making and a place to be brought into disability activism and culture.

Loree began her care collective in her twenties in Virginia as a survival strategy: the state's refusal to fund attendant care adequately (as is true most of the time with state social service) meant that the amount of money she got to pay attendants was below minimum wage. And often, when she was able to hire an attendant with DHSS money, they were homophobic and unsupportive of Erickson when she was watching queer films or hanging out with other queer friends. In response, Erickson fired her attendants, had a meeting with her friends, and came up with the vision to experiment with collective friend-made care together.

Her care collective continued when she moved to Toronto, partially because of her lack of ability to access state-funded home

---

12   Elizabeth Sweeney, "Young, Hot, Queer & Crip: Sexing Up Disability Is a Way of Life for Loree Erickson," *Daily Xtra*, September 9, 2009, https://www.dailyxtra.com/young-hot-queer-crip-12141.

care attendants because of her not being a permanent resident. For the past fifteen years, her care collective has been filled with disabled and non-disabled friends and community members who work shifts each week to help her with dressing, bathing, and transferring. She doesn't have to do all the care work herself: she has friends who take on the admin work of emailing, scheduling, and training potential care shifters. When she travels away from her home base of Toronto to conferences, to lecture and teach workshops, or to visit friends and lovers, she or supporters ask, via Facebook and email, for people in that region to help and be part of her care team. In recent years, Loree and allies have planned small fundraisers to purchase adaptive equipment and compensate some care shifters who are poor/low income for their time and care work, especially as Loree gets older, and her community gets more disabled themselves.

Loree's care collective is not just a practical survival strategy to get her the care she needs; it's a site of community and political organizing, where many people learn about disability politics (both the theory and the nitty-gritty) in action for the first time. In one interview, she notes that upon moving to Toronto, her care collective became a more explicitly political space. "It was more like mobilizing a community. I was meeting new people, I was connecting with folks, and I started to see the ways that collective care functions as anti-ableism training for folks," she said. People were becoming radicalized around care and disability through participating in the collective. "It's not like I'm giving workshops or lectures from the bathroom, but you know, we're talking about both of our lives and so that's part of the way that the education happens."[13]

In Loree's care collective, her need for access is posited as something she both needs and deserves, and as a chance to build community, hang out with Loree, and have fun—not as a chore. This

---

13   Muna Mire and Mary Jean Hande, "'The Pace We Need to Go': Creating Care Culture," *Action Speaks Louder: OPIRG-Toronto's Field Manual for Those Who've Had Enough*, Fall 2013, 8–9.

is drastically different from most ways care is thought of in the world, as an isolated, begrudgingly done task that is never a site of pleasure, joy, or community building.

This is radical. It is a radical rewriting of what care means, of what disability means, taking anarchist ideas of mutual aid and crip-femming them out. I've shown people Loree's fundraising video for the collective, where shots of her transferring to the toilet with the help of a care shifter are interspersed with footage of her and care shifters trading gossip and dating advice over breakfast. After seeing the video, one participant in a workshop on care I gave said, "It's really mind-blowing for me to see someone accessing care that's very intimate, without shame, and with everyone laughing and having a good time."

Loree's care collective model is a deep possibility model, not a one-size-fits-all solution for everyone who needs care. Her collective working relies on her having access to a broad network of friends and acquaintances, a social and activist life where people know her and are interested in helping her out, something many people, especially sick, disabled, and mad people, are too socially isolated to be able to access. Although I admire her collective and have learned a lot from watching it, I also think about how there aren't a million collectives for low-income Black and brown autistic, physically disabled, or chronically ill people in Toronto. I think of the challenges myself and Black and brown friends and acquaintances have had finding people who are willing and able to do care for a week or a month, let alone years, especially when that care involves pain or mental health crises that may not have a resolution. I think about the ways Loree's willingness to offer emotional caregiving to her care shifters, her whiteness and extroversion and neurotypicality are factors that aid her in being able to access an abundance of care—factors not available to everyone.

I also think about the people I know who want and need the distance of having someone they don't know care for them. As a wheelchair-using, physically disabled Black femme friend of mine remarked to me, "I'm glad Loree's model works for her, but if someone drops me, if someone doesn't show up for a shift, I can die. I don't ever want to depend on being liked or loved by the community for the right to shit in my toilet when I want to."

I think that all of these things can be true at the same time. Loree's collective is still an incredibly important example of a crip-created way of accessing care that has made more worlds of care possible for myself and others to dream.

CREATING COLLECTIVE ACCESS DETROIT, JUNE 2010–JUNE 2012

We know that for many of us, access is on our minds when it comes to traveling, navigating the city, movement spaces, buildings, sidewalks, public transportation, rides, the air, the bathrooms, the places to stay, the pace, the language, the cost, the crowds, the doors, the people who will be there and so so so much more.

Would you like to be connected to a network of crips and our allies/comrades who are working together to create collective access?

What is collective access? Collective Access is access that we intentionally create collectively, instead of individually.

Most of the time, access is placed on the individual who needs it. It is up to you to figure out your own access or, sometimes, up to you and your care giver, personal attendant (PA) or random friend. Access is rarely weaved into a collective commitment and way of being; it is isolated and relegated to an afterthought (much like disabled people).

Access is complex. It is more than just having a ramp or getting disabled folks/crips into the meeting. Access is a constant process that doesn't stop. It is hard and even when you have help, it can be impossible to figure out alone.

We are working to create mutual aid between crips and beyond! ... We hope that together we can create a culture of collective access. We are just trying this out! would you like to join us in practicing what this could look like? do you have ideas? are you an ally/comrade who wants to help out or be on call?[14]

Creating Collective Access (CCA) was a crip[15]-femme-of-color-made piece of brilliance that came together in the summer of 2010. You can read much more about it at creatingcollectiveaccess.wordpress.com, but in my version of the story, CCA happened because three disabled queer Asian femmes were on a conference call to plan the workshops we were organizing at the 2010 Allied Media Conference (AMC) and US Social Forum (USSF)—an enormous social justice gathering bringing tens of thousands of people to Detroit to imagine a revolutionary future—and we were completely fucking stressed out about how we were going to survive those conferences.

This is a very common disability experience: getting ready to go travel to a conference and having your freak-out about how badly the whole thing will fuck up your body. Will the airport break your wheelchair? Will you get sick from a fragrance exposure? Will the accessible van or ASL promised in the conference material just not be there? Where will the food be, and is it stuff you can eat? Will you be 1,000% overstimulated

---

14   "Crips Visiting Detroit!" *Creating Collective Access*, June 2, 2010, https://creatingcollective access.wordpress.com/2010/06/02/crips-visiting-detroit.

15   "Crip" is a word used by many people in disabled communities as a fuck-you, in-your-face reclaimed word, short for cripple—similar to how queers have reclaimed the word "queer." Not everyone likes it or uses it; people have complex feeling about it, and it's not great for abled people to use it. Leroy Moore coined the term "Krip" to avoid using a term that also is the name of the Crip gang/street economic organization.

by thousands of people talking about intense things? What if you have a panic attack or suicidal ideation 2,000 miles away from home and your usual supporters' access hacks? In short, how will you negotiate the world away from the crip survival skills you have where you live? We're used to feeling that our disability experiences are private, embarrassing, and not to be spoken about—especially crips who may be working mostly in non-disabled social justice communities—and conference and travel bring those feelings on even more so.

But in 2010, some of us came together at a nascent moment of disability justice organizing. We came together as disabled queer and trans people of color, talking, sometimes haltingly, about our intersectional lives, and talking about what disability organizing would mean that didn't leave any part of ourselves behind. We were rooted in a ground of other disabled queer and trans people of color, who were finding each other through online portals like the Azolla Story (a closed online portal for disabled queer and trans people of color, through the cultural, political work of Sins Invalid and the Disability Justice Collective, through our own blogs and chance meetings in crip-of-color hallways, coming and going. And on that call, Stacey, Mia, and I had a profound moment of clarity. We didn't have to choose between handling our access needs on our own or crossing our fingers that the conference and the airlines would come through to take care of us. We could experiment in coming together and caring for each other. What would it be like to create a space that centered Black and brown disabled people, that was led by disabled queer femmes of color, where instead of able-bodied people begrudgingly "helping" us, we were doing it for ourselves? We didn't know, but we knew it would be the polar opposite of so much existing disabled spaces that were dominated by white crips and their casual and overt racism, so much mainstream space where we were always on hold with access services. We didn't know what we were doing, and we knew what we were doing. We knew we were creating something revolutionary.

So we did it, and we did it quick, in the last three weeks before we had to go to Detroit—threw up a quick WordPress site asking for other sick and disabled queer, mostly Black and brown, people to find us, for us to find each other. We knew we couldn't create access for thousands of people, but we wanted to see what we could do with the resources we had.

And it worked: sick and disabled queer people of color found us, through email and Facebook posts and friends of friends, and, once we got there, through running into us on-site. It came together in that effortless-feeling way that happens sometimes when something's time has come. There was so much creativity, hustle, and fun—and disabled queer of color brilliance. One member of CCA drove up from North Carolina to Detroit with two other disabled POC and her personal care attendant in her wheelchair-accessible van. That van legally fits four people, but I have photos of thirteen crips crammed into it and driving through Detroit, laughing our asses off. We shared information about why fragrance-free body care products are important and shared the actual products, especially those for Black and brown hair and skin, with each other, including with people who'd never heard of "fragrance-free" before but were down if it meant we were able to be together. We booked a few accessible dorm suites so we could sleep and hang out with each other.

CCA was one of the first places I ran into what I would later call cross-disability solidarity, and more than that, the reality of our different disabilities not being a liability, that there could be ways we supported each other. One person selectively used some "poor, cute cripple" skills to charm the dorm staff and get them to unlock the fourth-floor kitchen so we could cook and store groceries. One neurodivergent person who didn't have mobility problems walked a mile to the closest restaurant to load up someone else's spare manual wheelchair with our shawarma orders and walked the food back to everyone who couldn't walk that far.

Being less isolated helped us make group demands of the AMC that were effective because they came from collective disabled power, not just one individual crip writing a request on a registration form. The AMC ordered in fragrance-free soap for the washrooms because Detroit back then didn't have any supermarkets, let alone one that stocked Dr Bronner's unscented. The relationships and collective power we built also helped us survive the USSF, which had some major access challenges (like, no wheelchair-accessible shuttle, even though it was on all the promo material, and when we called to ask where it was, the person we talked to was like, "Can you come to the conference site and ask about the shuttle?" and didn't quite get it when we were like, "No, we can't, because we can't physically get there"). I remember someone texting, "I am spooning out, I need crip love" from where they were passed out at one end of the conference center, and all of us getting there as fast we could, and them saying that just watching us walk and roll up made all the difference.

We didn't just survive the conference—we made powerful community. Committed to leaving no one behind, we rolled through the conference in a big, slow group of wheelchair users, cane users, and slow-moving people. Instead of the classic able-bodied conference experience most of us were used to, where able-bodied people walked at their able-bodied rate and didn't notice we were two blocks behind, or nowhere, we walked as slow as the slowest person and refused to abandon each other. People got out of the way. Instead of going out to inaccessible party sites, we chose to stay in, and ate and shared about our disabled lives. For some of us, it was our first time doing that. People cried, flirted, and fell in love.

CCA changed everyone who was present for it and a lot of people who just heard about it. It was just four days, but people went home to their communities transformed. We were no longer willing to accept isolation, or a tiny bit of access, or being surrounded by white disabled folks as the only kind of disability community we could access, or being forgotten. We talked about how it had been for us to be with each other. We threw queer disabled femme of color brunches that were maybe just us and the three other sick and disabled femmes of color we knew, but we sat in bed and talked and talked about our lives. We tried out starting crip hangouts and zines and performance nights. We started thinking about what it would mean to have our own care collectives, on a permanent basis. We came back less willing to accept ableism from conferences and community spaces, because we knew it could be different—and if CCA could happen in someplace with scarce physical resources like Detroit, it could happen anywhere. Being part of that wild pack of slowness, talking tentatively about our disabled lives in ways we'd never said out loud before, changed everyone's lives.

AN ASIDE: STORY THREE: THE CRASH-AND-BURN EMERGENCY MODEL

In many able-bodied activist communities—QTBIPOC and mostly-white punk—I've been a part of, I've been witness to another form of care web that is very different from the ones I've written about so far. They're the emergency-response care webs that happen when someone able-bodied becomes temporarily or permanently disabled, and their able-bodied network of friends springs into action. When the friend gets hit by a car when they're on their bike or gets pneumonia, there are emails and calls and care calendars set up, and (mostly able-bodied) people show up to the hospital. (Mostly able-bodied) people cook food and throw benefits. There's a sense of urgency! Purpose! Action! OMG, someone is sick! We must come together as a community to help them. (Many disabled people roll their eyes at this moment: *Wow, when it's your mountain-climbing friend who gets hit riding their bike, you care, huh? For me and the other folks who are always disabled, not so much, huh?*)

The urgent care calendar care web lasts for a few weeks, a month.

And then ... people trickle off. People think that the person's all better. It isn't a fun cause of the moment anymore. People think: *Wow, you're still disabled?*

These models have a lot to learn from disability justice models of centering sustainability, slowness, and building for the long haul. They tend to come from people who don't know, well, that disabled people or community or activism, um, exists. Since they don't know (or have been firmly ignoring) that we exist, they often reinvent the wheel(chair). I'm not the only crip who's felt bitter when I've seen calls for benefits and care earnestly sent out for someone who's been able-bodied up to that point and now has an acute, sudden need, when I've watched myself and my friends who have chronic disabilities, have been disabled since birth or live with chronic physical illness or dance with madness/mental health, struggle to get responses to our everyday and acute asks for care and support.

These emergency-response care webs often really fall apart when and if the person they're for becomes disabled in a long-term way, and the members realize that the "issue" isn't an individual problem that their buddy has—that beyond needing care, their friend is being impacted by the ableism of both the everyday world and much queer and activist space. Clubs they used to hang with aren't wheelchair accessible (they notice for the first time); fighting with insurance companies and the access van take hours. Huh! Is this a thing? The emails start coming in to the one crip they know: "Hey, do you know where so and so can find accessible housing? Seems like it's kind of hard to find." It's not that I don't want folks to access what they need—but I also have to roll my eyes that these folks are noticing ableism for the first time. I want them to understand that the struggles their friend is facing are not new or unique to them, that although I'll usually share my knowledge, so many of us have been using (limited) spoons[16] to fight these fights for a long time.

If these care webs are going to keep working, a paradigm shift needs to occur in those friends' heads. They need to see the disabled people they've blanked out on listening to for years when we've been trying to talk about access or our lives. (An apology might be cool, too.) They need to understand that their friend isn't a special cripple, cooler than the rest—that the problems they're facing aren't individual ones but systemic struggles that face all crips and need collective solutions. They need to ask themselves why they have systematically refused to value or take in what disabled folks around them have been and are saying. They need to listen and learn from the care work and skills disability communities have been doing for years—and maybe offer some compensation for that knowledge. Or at least say thank you.

STORY FOUR: CCA BAY AREA

In the fall of 2010, some of us who'd been in Detroit came back to the Bay Area where we lived or moved there for the first time. And it occurred to us: Why didn't we try and do something similar here? What would it mean to take the temporary experiment in crip-of-color–made access that had worked so beautifully during the four to ten days we'd be in Detroit to our homeplaces, in a long-term way?

We dove right into the modest, wildly ambitious plan of attempting

---

16   "Spoons" is slang created by sick and disabled communities to describe units of energy and capacity, specifically within a sick and disabled context of having a limited amount of energy because of chronic illness or disability (thus having to make decisions about which tasks to do and which to let slide, moving at a slower pace/"on crip time," etc.). The concept was created by Christine Miserandino in her essay "The Spoon Theory," posted on her website, *But You Don't Look Sick.* In her essay, a chronically ill woman attempting to describe what it's like to live with chronic illness pulls out a handful of spoons and uses them as units of energy, relating what it's like to have to carefully count how much energy you expend on daily tasks many abled people take for granted.

to create a Bay Area care collective by and for disabled queer and trans people of color.

We came together with a lot of hope and a ton of longing, a longing for a community we had been wanting for most of our lives. We came together with so much need and so much fear, like icebergs, where most of the mass lies below the surface.

When we sat down at our very first meeting, I thought I knew exactly how it was going to go. When I thought about what I might need in terms of disability care and support, I could name it right away: I could sure use some help driving my best friend to acupuncture and the grocery store and the mosque twice a week—I loved helping them, but between supporting them, supporting myself, and working two to three jobs, plus working on two or three unpaid collectives that were each like part-time jobs, I was exhausted. And, in a smaller tone of voice that didn't reach outside my head, *I could use folks who could help me do some stuff too.*

This project turned out to be a little more complicated than I'd thought it would. Everyone had a lot of questions. Should CCA Bay be open to white folks or just POC? Just crips or non-disabled QTBIPOC allies? Some argued that some of us had white crips in our "pods" of people we shared care with already, so it wouldn't make sense to exclude them. Other folks felt strongly that white disabled people always dominated crip space and did not want to risk creating a space where we would have to fight to continue to center people of color. Some felt that including non-disabled BIPOC folks could help develop seed organizers who could work to make the non-disabled QTBIPOC community less ableist.

But before we jumped into Google calendar, one member pulled out a flip chart. She said that before we did anything we needed to talk what would allow us to give and receive care. Most of us, she pointed out, had received shitty care, abusive care, care with strings attached. Most of us, she guessed, would want to give care, and then shrug and say, "I don't know, I'm fine" when asked what we needed. We went around: What made it possible for us to receive care? What was bound up with that act of reception? Under what conditions could we be vulnerable?

These, it turned out, were very deep and necessary questions. Hard to answer ones. The crip $64,000 questions. That friend was right: all of us were eager to offer care; receiving care, not so much. It was so much easier to offer care to other people than to ask for what we needed, for so many reasons. Many of us had been raised as immigrants and/or women or femmes of color to always jump up and feed people first, do all the dishes, and help without being asked, while serving ourselves last. For many of us, care had been something that was forced on us—something abusive family members or teachers or health care workers did, whether we liked it or not. Or care had been something it wasn't safe to say that we needed—because there was no care out there for us, no health care, no therapist, no parent with time, no safe parent who actually cared. Maybe as disabled people, if we wanted to have any kind of independence, we had to deny that we needed any help at all—in order to stay in mainstreamed classes, go to college, or date, we had to say that we didn't have any needs. I can remember my mother clearly telling me in high school, when I first thought I might be neurodivergent—it was decades before I would know that word, but I was still really fucking clear that my brain and cognition and my ability to navigate space were very different from most people around me—that it was unsafe for me to say that I might need a tutor—tutors and accommodations, newly allowed under the brand new ADA, were for the rich white boys; I just had to be twice as smart and keep up if I wanted to get a scholarship. I couldn't afford to look "stupid."

And finally, some of our needs were so vulnerable, so embarrassing, so complicated to ask for that it was much easier to just not admit we needed them. In that go round, when I silently thought, *I could use some help too,* one of the first things I thought of was that when I was sick, I often needed help with housework—making my bed and doing dishes, chores, and laundry, buying groceries, and cooking food. But as a working-class femme, raised by an ex-waitress mom who taught me to always bus my own table, and as someone who'd cleaned houses for a living, I had a strong working-class ethic about always doing my own housework. I couldn't imagine asking one of my friends to clean my toilet or do my dishes without feeling like an asshole—even though I regularly and happily did chores for friends when they were sick.

We met an average of twice a week for a year. A lot of our time was spent building relationships, hanging out, and supporting each other in different ways, from physical care to emotional care during breakups. And we faced some challenges that many groups like ours have faced and will face again. We realized that even though we were all queer and trans disabled people of color, we didn't automatically know each other's access needs cross-disability. People who were physically disabled didn't automatically understand the needs of folks who were Mad, and vice versa. Sometimes, we thought of those misunderstanding as betrayals, instead of opportunities to own our mistakes or ask each other to teach us.

Mia Mingus's often-quoted words, from her essay of the same name about committing to crip community, "Wherever you are is where I want to be"[17] got put to the test when access needs weren't complementary and we couldn't physically be in the same space. When someone needed help moving out of their house up two flights of stairs,

---

17   Mia Mingus, "Wherever You Are Is Where I Want to Be: Crip Solidarity," *Leaving Evidence*, May 3, 2010, https://leavingevidence.wordpress.com/2010/05/03/where-ever-you-are-is-where-i-want-to-be-crip-solidarity/, accessed July 2, 2018.

even though the call for help said, "Come if you can help move and lift boxes! Come by if you just want to lend moral support! Bring food to share" (suggesting that helping physically move boxes, bringing food, and offering moral support were all equally legit ways of supporting)—but if I was too fatigued to get out of bed and too broke to bring food, did that mean that I wasn't being a good community member? We were running into a similar challenge Loree had once talked about with an earlier care web she'd been involved in: What happens when chronically ill folks—who often have fatigue, lack of physical strength, and a need to shift and cancel schedules as we get sick—try to assist physically disabled folks, who often need folks to be able to lift heavy things, and who may have pretty scheduled lives (e.g., chair users who have PCA care shifts when they pee scheduled every four to six hours)? We weren't always great at sitting with those contradictions with kindness and curiosity, an "Okay, that didn't work—what would?

Often, instead, we experienced the places where interdependence didn't just magically work out as betrayal, letting each other down. We had so many hopes for each other, so much belief that we could be everything to each other, effortlessly and automatically, through shared identity. And we'd been betrayed so many times before, by white disabled people and non-disabled people in our lives, so we hoped that since we'd finally, finally found that beloved BIPOC sick and disabled community, we'd never fuck up (or be tired), always know the right thing to do, and be able to do it. It turned out that, like every time I've come together with people I've shared an identity with, there was bliss and also heartbreak when we assumed that that bliss would be easy and forever.

As romham of RAMP Vancouver writes:

> If interdependency is in our DNA, what does it mean when
> we fall out of whack with it? How do we handle the realities

of our bodies and minds that need what they need when they need it? What does it mean when I can't support you in the ways you're supporting me? Does interdependency mean we do the same for one another at all times, as though there's even such a thing as "the same" when it comes to this stuff? Is it a gentle ebb and flow? What if my ebb will never match your flow? What if it's sometimes a torrential downpour and one of us is drowning? What do we do then?[18]

There were more questions. Like, what happened when some of us could hang together more because we had fewer mobility needs—we could make it into a car, could deal with exposures—and some of us couldn't? How did we make things feel fair when some of us got tired and sick and needed to cancel, and others—maybe folks who practiced "sucking it up" and working through pain more, maybe just folks who didn't have pain and fatigue—were left feeling like they were doing all the work? What about those of us who felt more comfortable going to non-disabled events together so got to spend that time and get that visibility, and those of us who felt more overwhelmed or had more anxiety about being stared at?

And, maybe the biggest disabled community question of all: What happens when a lot of people who have always been the only one, are no longer the only disabled queer of color in the room? How does that affect how we work together, build community, and work out conflict? Sometimes, because we were used to being the only revolutionary crip fighting ableism in a sea of able-bodied obliviousness, it was hard for us to hear that we weren't always right, to understand differences of opinion or approach or experience as other than wrong, or attack, or threat.

---

18   "What Happens When We Can't Live Interdependency All the Time?" *Radical Access Mapping Project*, November 9, 2015, https://radicalaccessiblecommunities.wordpress.com/2015/11/09/what-happens-when-it-feels-like-we-cant-live-interdependency-all-the-time/.

After a year, our group broke up, from all of these pressures and hard spots and a web of interpersonal conflict. It was a hard breakup. I felt like my dream sick and disabled QTBIPOC crew had fallen apart, that a community I had passionately believed in and given much of my limited energy to had failed.

I didn't know that one group falling apart didn't have to mean that was it—for the idea of building a care web, for the movement. I wish we could've known that the struggles we hit weren't failures or signs of how inadequate we were but incredibly valuable learnings. I wish I'd known then what I do now—that all this stuff is the $6 million crip question, that we were by far not the only disabled queers to struggle with them, and that our struggle to figure these questions out is at the heart of our movement work. CCA is another worthy, imperfect model in my body's archive, one I build on as I build care in my life now.

STORY FIVE: AN ONGOING, VIRTUAL CARE WEB: SICK AND DISABLED QUEERS

Disabled Mizrahi genderqueer writer and organizer Billie Rain started Sick and Disabled Queers (SDQ), a Facebook group for well, sick, and disabled queers, in 2010. Billie started SDQ as an experiment in building an online community open to all sick and disabled queer people that would center sick and disabled queer people of color and other folks who had traditionally been marginalized from mainstream disability rights spaces, that would also be accessible to the many sick and disabled queers who were isolated, homebound, or had limited energy or ability to travel physically to an in-person meeting. Mostly, Billie wanted a place where a lot of sick and disabled queer people could hang out in bed, online, and chat with each other. Over the eight years of its existence, SDQ blew up into a virtual, North America–wide community that both offered a hell of a lot of practical care and support—shared knowledge about diseases and doctors and disability hearings, people witnessing each other and fundraising for rent and medical bills and accessible vans—and became a locus of disability justice thinking, relationship building, and organizing.

It is impossible for me separate the care work SDQ members did from the theories we made, from how we shared tools, wrote poetry, and created friendships. SDQ folks regularly mailed each other meds and extra inhalers and adaptive equipment. We shared, when asked, information about what treatments worked for us and what didn't and tips for winning a disability hearing. We crowdsourced money for folks who needed to replace stolen wheelchairs, detox their houses, get living expenses together for rehab, or get out of unsafe housing situations. People sent care packages and organized visit teams for members they might never have met in person who were in the hospital, rehab, or the psych ward. We cocreated an evolving, amazing cross-disability best practices/community guidelines document that helps folks learn about the disabilities that aren't ours—from captioning videos to neurodivergent communication styles. At its height, it was everything good that social media made possible—instant connection with a million people with shared identities and interests, who could listen to you when you were in crisis or answer a disability question that no one near you knew the answer to. It was a structure that broke two of the biggest barriers most disabled people face—isolation and shame.

SDQ felt like a hot spot of disability justice in practice. Some of the smartest DJ thought happened here, and mostly, it felt free of "activist stardom" but filled with collective disabled intelligence. Instead of a few Special Crips, it felt like a place where a lot of folks, often especially folks who were deeply isolated and excluded from systemic power and the world, got to think and talk with each other, take and share pictures of ourselves in bed, share tips about hypermobility and sex, diagnose each other way faster than the free clinic could—and also ask big questions about disability, art, sex, activism, and life. SDQ at its best functioned as a big, sustainable, pretty damn cross-accessible care web powered by members who were homebound, not working a lot, isolated, on disability, and who had time to throw down support, prayers, and connection via text, the internet, or phone. Because the format was text based, it was Deaf accessible and accessible to folks for whom voice and in-person communication is hard. It was and is a more challenging/less accessible format for folks who are working, anxious, or overwhelmed by a lot of internet, or EMF sensitive so that being on the computer is hard or impossible.

SDQ had a community value of people responding how they can, as they can, with no shame if they didn't have capacity. SDQ is also a model of what we mean when we try to explain that disabled people know how to do sustainability. SDQ was inherently very sustainable because it wasn't just you trying to ask your crew of six local people for help—you could reach out to thousands of people across the world, and someone would always be up, someone would always have cash or capacity or energy to talk you through whatever it was. SDQ grew from a community with one moderator to one with six, so there was always someone to step in if someone else was sick or spooned out. SDQ felt like a living example of what sustainable organizing looks like, led by people who are pushed out of 99% of able-bodied mainstream activism and are told that we aren't capable of doing any kind of organizing or political activity.

I remember a heated debate on SDQ where a new member said they liked the space, but it "didn't seem like there was much activism going on here." People got really heated. We talked passionately about how what we were doing on SDQ—the talking and the meds-sharing and the scheming and the life support—absolutely counted as activism, was a way we were transforming traditional notions of what activism was to make it over in our own cripped-out images. And that without the life support we were giving each other, we wouldn't be able to stay alive to do activism, or life, at all.

CARE FUTURES

As I write this, Trump is in his second year. We've withstood his government's attempts to destroy the ADA, the Affordable Care Act's access to health care for disabled and sick people, and Medicaid's funding of paid home attendant care. Everyone I know is a mix of on edge, permanently wondering what shit will hit the fan next, trying not to be stuck in reactivity and panic, and sometimes, absurdly hopeful and passionate about building the futures we need.

I am ten years in to these wild experiments with collective access and care, and I am both grateful for the stories under my belt and full of the knowledge of how much I still don't know. I continue to live a life supported by a practice of being able to call on kin in emergencies and everyday need and being able to respond to need. I am a veteran of many emergency care circles and GoFundMes that have come together when someone is facing a disability crisis—eviction, medical bills, emergencies, mental health crisis. I know some things about how to organize a circle of people who can offer care, stop by with food, send money, and text people back.

Yet as I move forward in this life of creating and receiving care, I am continually impressed by how we find ways to keep each other alive when the state is fucked, and community can be fucked and inadequate too. I love seeing how friends and strangers seem to be more and more used to crowdfunding care and setting up care shift Google docs. I also see the burnout and exploitation of often femme and disabled labor that happens, and also what happens when people plain run out of energy, money, and time. I think about the needs I have that I am still too ashamed to let anyone see, let alone take care of.

I also think about friends and strangers who have plenty of needs but not enough friends or strangers willing and able to come through to care for them. The community is not a magic utopia, just like our families weren't, and we don't all just magically love each other, or even like each other, let alone agree on every political issue. I think about people I know who are mean or angry or bitter or "hard to like"—and disabled—and how that confluence is not a surprise or an accident, because many of us are indeed in a shitty mood, mean, or bitter from withstanding decades of ableism and the isolation that it brings. I think about the people I know who I don't want to die lying in their own piss, but I don't want to be the one who changes their diaper either. I think about the things I still can't ask friends to help me with—cleaning the house when it's incredibly nasty after I've been in pain for weeks, dealing with shit or blood. I think about my friend's statement that she shouldn't have to rely on being liked or loved to get care.

I recently realized I was hitting caregiving burnout—something I was familiar with as a concept but never thought would happen to me—with a loved one after many months of chronic illness and mental health crisis on both our parts. After a Google search connected me with a caregivers' website for my county and I sent an email, I got a nice phone call back from someone from who told me that we would be eligible for twenty-four hours of emergency respite care—someone would be paid by the county to show up, pick up the meds, do the dishes, cook some food, and listen. She tactfully said, "Many people find they have an easier time with someone who is being paid, well, to do the work, coming in and helping than asking a friend to clean and cook." When I told my friend that this existed, not only did they agree, they exclaimed, "How come all our friends aren't using this, instead of just burning each other out?" I know the answers—shame, lack of access to the web, thinking that it doesn't exist or the actuality that it really doesn't exist or we won't be eligible or we'll have to jump through rings of fire to get it. And it made me see more possibilities.

I don't think there is any one single answer to the need for care. I just want, to echo my friend Dori, more care, more of the time. I want us to dream mutual aid in our postapocalyptic revolutionary societies where everyone gets to access many kinds of care—from friends and internet strangers, from disabled community centers, and from some kind of non-fucked-up non-state state that would pay caregivers well and give them health benefits and time off and enshrine sick and disabled autonomy and choice. I want us to keep dreaming and experimenting with all these big, ambitious ways we dream care for each other into being.

SOME TOOLS AND PITFALLS TO WATCH OUT FOR, FOR FOLKS DREAMING CARE WEBS

Crips supporting crips! Only! Ever! Crip-on-crip support is awesome! Often, after a lifetime of ableist able-bodied people providing shitty or abusive care and assuming that we're not able to do anything ourselves, disabled people caring for each other can be a place of deep healing. Many, if not most of us, have good reasons not to trust that able-bodied people will actually get it, will actually come through on their promises of care or support. Lots of disabled folks I know who are well versed in this experience also understand that it's mostly only other sick and disabled folks who actually show up for each other. We can be projectile vomiting and we'll still send you a supportive text from the side of the toilet.

However, moving together as disabled people, in my mind, has some important caveats. Solidarity with other crips also means the realities of an inaccessible world and cross-ability access. If I am chronically ill and don't have the energy/strength to lift you onto the toilet, that doesn't mean I am a bad ally. There's also the reality that sometimes we all need care, simultaneously. I've often seen crip-only spaces fill with feelings of betrayal and hopelessness when we cannot fulfill some of our friends' needs. Instead, I believe it's possible to build a model of experimenting and seeing how it works out, then adjusting. We can try, knowing we may fail and things may turn out to be more complicated than we expected.

I also think that recruiting non-disabled folks who actually have their shit together (or can be trained to) can be a great option for some care. And what about paying some folks, in cash or work/ skill trade, some of the time for spoons or energy-demanding labor? How about valuing a system of people contributing as they can, not necessarily "equally" or "always"?

Assuming that as crips we intrinsically understand each other's access needs, or that access intimacy (even when we have the same kind of disability) is automatic. Or that even if we really get each other's shit at first, our needs don't change over time.

Not paying attention to the gendered/raced/classed dynamics of care—a.k.a., are the poor and working-class disabled femmes doing all the work all the time? Care is feminized and invisibilized labor. Care is something that many (not all) poor/working-class folks do like breathing—we got time! It's just the right thing to do, right? What's going on with race and entitlement? Who feels comfy asking? Are the white queers, the pretty queers, the middle-class, relatively happy, skinny, normal queers getting much care? How many masculine-gendered people have I cared the ass off for, with no reciprocity? Talk about this stuff! It's really important! Disrupt it! Get the masc, pretty, abled people to put in time!

Doing all the admin work yourself! So often I've seen sick and disabled folks do everything—all the caregiving, all the resource buying, and all the emailing and filing. Get some eager able-bodied person to manage the damn calendar!

Assuming there is one right way to do "it"—it being the ways we offer or organize care—and that a way that works for a while won't change. The circle of six people who come together at first may not be able to keep doing everything forever. The one person who was so great at doing the admin/organization end of things may get really sick of doing it, especially if they're holding all the notes in their head. Build capacity. Share the tools someplace everyone can access them. Switch out roles. Plan for people giving care to have our own crises. Having only one person with the skills and capacity to coordinate stuff is a recipe for burnout.

Assuming that care webs have to be huge or that someone else somewhere is the "expert." We're so used to disabled care being professionalized, to assuming that medical and therapeutic professionals are the only ones qualified to intersect with our terrifying bodies. But the first CCA was created on three weeks' notice. Collective care, like transformative justice, can be so many things—a "crip your hangout" hangout, an ASL meetup, a Lotsa Helping Hands calendar, a hangout where I bring you food and we smoke high-CBD weed.

Sometimes it's not perfect. Often, disabled folks are (surprise) isolated. Some people have a big community to draw on; many of us don't. But just like some access is better than none, some (good) care can be better than none—and can be built on.

QUESTIONS TO ASK YOURSELF AS YOU START A CARE WEB OR COLLECTIVE, AND KEEP ASKING

- What is the goal of your care web? Who needs care? What kind?
- Who's in it? What are their roles: caregiver, care receiver, both, admin person, fundraiser?
- How are you resisting the charity model in your work?
- What are best practices that allow the people receiving care to receive care well?
- What are best practices that allow the people offering care to offer care well?

- What physical tools (A van? Scent-free cleanser? A car? A smartphone?) do you need to make the access work? What money or other resources do you need to make it happen?
- How will you celebrate and make it fun?
- How will you build in time off and times when people are sick and you need a plan B?
- What meeting structure do you need to check in, talk through issues, and keep things on track?
- Are you building in ways for disabled folks to offer care, instead of assuming that only able-bodied people are the "care-ers"?
- What's your plan for dealing with conflict when it happens?
- How are you going to document your work? Do you need a place to keep receipts, a log of who does what hours?
- Do you have a plan for checking in and making sure funky dynamics aren't creeping into your care? This could be anything from pity, martyrdom, guilt, or difficulty negotiating boundaries to the ways gender dynamics (women or femme people doing more care than masculine people and receiving less, expectations that many genders of people are supposed to "have it all together"), race dynamics (universalization of white experience, racism creeping in when Black or brown people are doing cleaning or physical care for white folks), class dynamics, whorephobia, internalized ableism, or cross-disability dynamics (for example, the differences between the experiences of more visibly/apparently disabled folks and those whose disabilities are invisiblized). (These are just some examples, not an exhaustive list.) It helps to view these issues coming up as part of the work and to have a proactive, scheduled time to check in about them.

CRIP EMOTIONAL INTELLIGENCE

Black queer femme writer Kim Katrin Milan created the phrase "femme science"[19] to mean femme skills, technologies, and intelligences. For me, it was revolutionary to hear someone state that femmes had actual, particular skills, talents, sciences, and cultures. I'm not sure when I started hearing and using the terms "crip skills" or "crip science"— probably roughly around the same time. But it meant something. It meant something to name and talk about all the crip skills I was seeing and learning that I and other disabled folks had. It meant something because, well, the deficiency model by which most people view disability only sees disabled people as a lack, a defect, damaged good, in need of cure. The idea that we have cultures, skills, science, and technology runs counter to all of that. In a big way.

Naming that also means having to field some able-bodied blank stares. Able-bodied people are shameless about really not getting it that disabled people could know things that the abled don't. That we have our own cultures and histories and skills. That there might be something that they could learn from us.

But we do, and we are. So here are some things I've noticed as hallmarks of crip emotional intelligence, skills we use within our cultures and with each other.

---

19   Kim Katrin Milan, "Femme Science & Community Based Research, presented at the Allied Media Conference, 2013," https://prezi.com/bkpfroriyfuz/femme-science-community-based-research/, accessed May 28, 2018.

- Crip emotional intelligence means not taking it personally sometimes, when another disabled person is short with you, is fumbling for words, is frustrated. Instead, you might assume that they just threw up for eight hours, have been fighting suicide for a week, have cellulitis in one of their legs again, have five giant fibroids and are struggling to decide what treatments to try. I'm not talking about excusing verbal abuse; I'm talking about the ways in which we cut each other slack. I'm talking about the ways we start from the assumption that someone might be dealing with a lot of pain, or facing a seven-layer cake of ableism and impairments, or struggling to use verbal language. I'm talking about the gift we give each other of seeing what the able-bodied imagination refuses to see: that sick, disabled, Mad, Deaf, and neurodivergent lives, and the stress we hold from places where ableism rubs up against them 'til they chafe, are normal. This is the norm, the default we assume is happening, rather than being oddballs who don't fit into an abled norm and have to apologize for it. Crip emotional intelligence is also not always losing it when someone doesn't use precisely the right word. It's knowing the difference between someone being a fucker and someone who has a brain injury, aphasia, extreme social isolation, or just didn't go to Oberlin.
- It's also figuring out how to communicate using smaller words, not academic words, different words than you just tried, writing. It's waiting for someone to be done finishing spelling out a sentence on their augmented communication device before responding. It's using text. It is not assuming that audist and academic ways of communicating are the smartest or the best.
- It's not assuming. Anything. It's always asking: if you can touch, what you call your body or your sick, what you need, if you even want suggestions for your issue or if you just want listening. It's

understanding that each disabled person is the expert on their own body/mind.

- Crip emotional intelligence is understanding isolation. Deeply. We know what it's like to be really, really alone. To be forgotten about, in that way where people just don't remember you've ever been out, at meetings and parties, in the social life of the world. How being isolated, being shunned, being cut off from the social world of community is terrifying because you know that it can literally kill you. And that being alone also does not always have to be killing; it can also be an oasis of calm, quiet, low stimulation, and rest.

- Crip emotional intelligence is not taking it personally when someone cancels and continuing to invite them to things. To not forget them.

- Is not shaming someone for precut vegetables or wet wipes or going to the drive-through or using a car. Including an SUV, because it's big enough to fit a chair.

- Is understanding that disabled people have a full-time job managing their disabilities and the medical-industrial complex and the world—so regular expectations about work, energy, and life can go right out the window.

- Is understanding the terror of ODSP or SSDI reviews, the food stamp office lines, that you never miss a specialist appointment, that going to the doctor is not usually the first response, that if you leave your disabled parking pass somewhere it's incredibly stressful, that so much of your money goes to pills or co-pays or therapy or supplements.

- Is noticing and showing respect for all the ways we push ourselves past our spoons all the time—when someone counsels someone in the middle of panic or blows their wrist spoons typing out resources. It understanding that we are in a constant dance of negotiating how to work while disabled or sick or in pain.

- Is sharing resources and showing up, and having a spoken or unspoken rule that acknowledges that you both (the two crips in the situation) have stuff going on. You will offer what you can. You will stop when you have to. You will accept "no" to your offer without taking it personally.

- Is the ability to read someone's face, body language, and energy to tell that they are in pain or struggling. Is being fluent in the skills of noticing pain, fatigue, overwhelm, and trigger.

- Is knowing that phrases like "Hope you feel better soon!" or "Awww, that succcccks!" are dirty words when they come from abled people after you describe your disability.

- Is understanding that if you find an accessible way to exercise for your body, that's great. But if you spent the day on the couch—because there is no way of exercising that doesn't cause pain, or because you can't move much, or because you just want to—that's just fine too. Understanding that it's a sacred task to not shame each other for being in bed in a world where completing the Ironman or going to Zumba is shoved down everyone's throats with no understanding of how "healthy" can hurt.

- Is understanding that beds are worlds. Houses are worlds. Cars are worlds.

- Is understanding that there are a million ways to be sexual (if one is sexual), and some of them live in phones, don't ever involve genitals, happen once a year. Is understanding that all movement is movement, and counts, including when someone can only move three fingers and part of their forehead. All sex is sex.

- Is understanding that when someone says, "I feel like shit/I'm feeling sick," the automatic reply shouldn't always be, "Oh, stay home/don't do it/let me do that for you!" That instead, you can say, "I'm sorry," without trying to fix it and say, "What feels possible today?"

- Is understanding that everything will break, everything will take longer than you think, the elevator will be broken at the BART station and Paratransit will be three hours late. And that these are not surprises. These are deliberate acts in a world that doesn't value or fund access.

- Is offering to do laundry. Is offering to do it again. Is knowing you will probably have to offer help a million times before another disabled person takes you up on it.
- Is offering what you can. Is asking if you can offer. Is saying when you can't.
- Is understanding that when someone does something themselves, even when it looks like it's full of struggle, that's not always them "being passive-aggressive." Sometimes, this is just us, hauling the groceries up the stairs, the way it looks like when we do that. Sometimes, we don't want to a pat on the head. Sometimes, we have learned not to depend on people who then fail to show up and complain about how hard it is to help a disabled person.
- Is knowing that offering miracle cures is a dirty word. Is knowing that cure is not mostly the point. Is knowing that our bodies don't need to be cured or fixed into normalcy to be valuable.
- Is tending to give each other the benefit of the doubt. We have been thrown away by so many people. We try not to throw each other away. No matter how unpopular or shitty the opinions expressed may be.
- Is knowing the algebra of pushing past and/or massaging your limits so that you can drive home, accompany someone at the hospital, perform a daily task, cook, eat. Is knowing that "Just do self-care!" is well meaning but totally inadequate. Is knowing we do more than we can all the time. Is knowing that "limits" is a negotiation.
- Is never assuming. Anything.

MAKING SPACE ACCESSIBLE IS AN ACT OF LOVE FOR OUR COMMUNITIES

Note: This piece was one of many pieces written in the lead-up to the 2010 US Social Forum, as we planned Creating Collective Access (CCA) in, I think, three weeks. This is one of those pieces that you pound out from bed, at two in the afternoon or one in the morning, when you hurt and you can't sleep, to serve a purpose.

I was asked to write something that would ask disabled people coming to CCA who didn't have chemical injuries to do the solidarity work of going fragrance-free for the gathering so that people whose disabilities meant that chemicals and fragrances made them sick would be able to attend. This was a particular, specific kind of access work, as part of the work involved my talking about fragrance and chemical access in a way that centered Black and brown people—to be specific, getting people to think of chemical access as not some weird shit only particularly annoying white vegans cared about but reframing it as something that Black and brown people have, due to everything from cleaning houses and working with pesticides to living in polluted cities, from having asthma to cancer. And to not only get people to reframe chemical disabilities form the whitewashed way they'd often been discussed but to provide a list of body and hair care products that were cheap, easy to get or make, and worked on Black and brown hair and skin. That last part became one of my most-used resources: "Fragrance-Free Femme of Color Genius" (formerly "Realness"), a compendium of products made with all my Virgo moon hyperfocus research skills.

But this piece picked up steam and got passed around in ways I hadn't expected. I guess writing about access as a form of radical solidarity called love hit a nerve.

When I think about access, I think about love.

I think that crip solidarity, and solidarity between crips and non(yet)-crips is a powerful act of love and I-got-your-back. It's in big things, but it's also in the little things we do moment by moment to ensure that we all—in all our individual bodies—get to be present fiercely as we make change.

Embedded in this is a giant paradigm shift. Our crip bodies aren't seen as liabilities, something that limits us and brings pity, or something to nobly transcend, 'cause I'm just like you. Our crip bodies are gifts, brilliant, fierce, skilled, valuable. Assets that teach us things that are relevant and vital to ourselves, our communities, our movements, the whole goddamn planet.

If I'm having a pain day and a hard time processing language and I need you to use accessible language, with shorter words and easiness about repeating if I don't follow, and you do, that's love. And that's solidarity. If I'm not a wheelchair user and I make sure I work with the non-disabled bottom-liner for the workshop to ensure that the pathways through the chairs are at least three feet wide, that is love and solidarity. This is how we build past and away from bitterness and disappointment at movements that have not cared about or valued us. When I've said this, some people have reacted in anger, saying that disabled folks shouldn't have to be loved to get access. They argue that we should simply have our rights under the law, as disabled citizens, respected. For me, this is an excellent example of where disability rights bumps against disability justice. A rights framework says that the ADA and other pieces of civil rights legislation give disabled "citizens" our rights: we simply state the law and get our needs met. Disability justice says: What if you're disabled and undocumented? What if you think the settler colonial nation we live in is a farce and a hallucination? What if you don't have money to sue an inaccessible business? What if the people giving you accommodations and access technology—or not—are not paid for by the state but part of your community?

I agree that our access to access and the world should not be predicated on desirability or popularity or approval of the able-bodied masses—or anyone. And I hold a deep place of respect for the ways so many of us have been denied access to love. But when I say the word "love," I mean something more cripped-out and weird than the traditional desirability politics many of us are forced to try to survive and live within.

I mean that when we reach for each other and make the most access possible, it is a radical act of love. When access is centralized at the beginning dream of every action or event, that is radical love. I mean that access is far more to me than a checklist of accessibility needs—though checklists are needed and necessary. I mean that without deep love and care for each other, for our crip bodyminds, an event can have all the fragrance-free soap and interpreters and thirty-six-inch-wide doorways in the world. And it can still be empty. I've been asked to do disability and access trainings by well-meaning organizations that want the checklists, the ten things they can do to make things accessible. I know that if they do those things, without changing their internal worlds that see disabled people as sad and stupid, or refuse to see those of us already in their lives, they can have all the ASL and ramps in the world, and we won't come where we're not loved, needed, and understood as leaders, not just people they must begrudgingly provide services for.

I mean that the sick and disabled spaces I have been in, been changed by, helped make, stumbled within at their best have been spaces full of deep love. And that deep love has been some of the most intense healing I've felt. It is a love that the medical-industrial complex and ableist society don't understand. It's why doctors scratch their heads and remark that I seem to be doing so well, and then stare blankly when I say that I have a lot of loving disabled community and it's what helps me. It took ten years to begin to not hate my bodymind. It took ten more to even begin to be able to ask for what I needed, matter-of-factly, without shame.

I mean more. I mean things like the radical notion that everyone deserves basic income, care, and access. Everyone. Including people you don't like. Including people who are not that likable. I can think of people who have, frankly, acted like assholes and hurt people in my life, or me. Some of them I have still sent twenty dollars, when I had it, to their Indiegogos when they got disabled and needed money for rent, food, housing, or to move to a more accessible apartment or city. Because nobody deserves to die or suffer from lack of access, even if they've been an asshole. I have seen some people doing the best DJ work possible, holding practices of, say, inviting everyone to their Friday night dinner—including people seen as cranky, unpopular, or difficult—because the most cripped-out folks were the most socially isolated and needed it the most.

Many of us who are disabled are not particularly likable or popular in general or amid the abled. Ableism means that we—with our panic attacks, our trauma, our triggers, our nagging need for fat seating or wheelchair access, our crankiness at inaccessibility, again, our staying home—are seen as pains in the ass, not particularly cool or sexy or interesting. Ableism, again, insists on either the supercrip (able to keep up with able-bodied club spaces, meetings, and jobs with little or no access needs) or the pathetic cripple. Ableism and poverty and racism mean that many of us are indeed in bad moods. Psychic difference and neurodivergence also mean that we may be blunt, depressed, or "hard to deal with" by the tenants of an ableist world.

And: I am still arguing for the radical notion that we deserve to be loved. As we are. As is.

At the risk of seeming like a Christian, or a Che Guevara poster, love is bigger, huger, more complex, and more ultimate than petty fucked-up desirability politics. We all deserve love. Love as an action verb. Love in full inclusion, in centrality, in not being forgotten. Being loved for our disabilities, our weirdness, not despite them.

Love in action is when we strategize to create cross-disability access spaces. When we refuse to abandon each other. When we, as disabled people, fight for the access needs of sibling crips. I've seen able-bodied organizers be confused by this. Why am I fighting so hard for fragrance-free space or a ramp, if it's not something I personally need?

When disabled people get free, everyone gets free. More access makes everything more accessible for everybody.

And once you've tasted that freedom space, it makes inaccessible spaces just seem very lacking that kind of life-saving, life-affirming love. Real skinny. Real unsatisfying. And real full of, well, hate.

Why would you want to be part of that?

So when you work to make spaces accessible, and then more accessible, know that you can come from a deep, profound place of love. And if you can't love us, or love yourself—know that the daily practice of loving self is intertwined with any safe room, accessible chairs, ramp. Both/and. When they are there, they show our bodies that we belong.

Love gets laughed at. What a weak, nonpolitical, femme thing. Love isn't a muscle or an action verb or a survival strategy. Bullshit, I say. Making space accessible as a form of love is a disabled femme of color weapon.

TORONTO CRIP CITY

A NOT-SO-BRIEF, INCOMPLETE PERSONAL HISTORY OF SOME MOMENTS IN TIME, 1997–2015

Toronto has a rich history of disabled organizing and community making by and for sick, disabled, Crazy, and Deaf queer and trans Black, Indigenous, and people of color (QTBIPOC). That organizing has taken place in a million ways—from street protests to Facebook fights, from kitchen-table conversations to envisioning what accessible sex parties would look like.

On the wall above my desk hangs a tattered, xeroxed flyer for a queer South Asian community event, sponsored by Desh Pardesh, Toronto's iconic radical South Asian festival. (Part of the reason I still have the flyer is because I had an under-the-table job flyering for the event series it was part of.) It's for a panel discussion on "community-based healing," and while it doesn't use the term "disability justice," it does feature three Filipina and South Asian speakers talking about madness in people of color communities, decolonizing yoga, and barriers faced by immigrants trying to access health care. Held in the Parkdale community library, a free, heavily used space that at the center of a Black and brown immigrant neighborhood filled with disabled people, it also proudly announces that it offers free on-site childcare, free tokens, and a wheelchair-accessible space. This workshop was *held in the year 2000*. Whenever someone ventures to say that giving a shit about and talking about disability and access are new things in our communities, I want to point to that damn flyer.

I realized while working on this essay that someone needs to write a book about this history because it's much bigger than one article could do justice to. There are a million more stories I could tell, and want to: the stories of Camp SIS (Camp Sisters in Struggle, a queer Indigenous women and women of color land project that also puts on shows that's been in Toronto and Ontario since the late '90s) insisting on ASL and access in their annual Pride shows and the presence of disabled queer women of color at those shows and their organizing collective; Unapologetic Burlesque offering radically deep access, from ASL to live captioning of every single song lyric to greeters welcoming those who might be isolated or socially anxious; organizing by Mad people of color in the 2010s; the queer ASL classes that many Toronto hearing and Deaf QTBIPOC began taking in 2011, leading to some combating of audism within hearing SDQTBIPOC and QTBIPOC communities; Accessexable, a small collective of Toronto-based disabled queers, trying to create crip-made broadly accessible sex parties in Toronto in the mid-2000s after years of the Pussy/Pleasure Palace, a popular Toronto queer sex party, being held in an inaccessible play space.

These stories didn't make it in here. This is a partial, incomplete history. Yet I believe, like many partial, incomplete histories, it is still of use. I am not a trained historian, but I am, like many people, someone who remembers and fights to remember as an act of both resistance and changing the future, who has sought to record my stories and the stories of my communities when I write. In writing this essay, one of my models was Joan Nestle—working-class Jewish femme writer and teacher, disabled cancer survivor, bar dyke from the Bronx. In books like *A Restricted Country* and *The Persistent Desire: A Femme-Butch Reader,* and in pieces like "Lesbians and Prostitutes: A Historical Sisterhood," Nestle recorded the working-class femme, sex worker, and queer and trans histories of herself and her community—as personal moments of memory, encounters in doorways, buried stories dug up. I also thought of Mia Mingus's iconic disability justice blog *Leaving Evidence*, where she says of disabled queer people of color, "We must leave evidence. Evidence that we were here, that we existed, that we survived and loved and ached. Evidence of the wholeness we never felt and the immense sense of fullness we gave to each other. Evidence of who we were, who we thought we were, who we never should have been. Evidence for each other that there are other ways to live—past survival; past isolation."[20] In recording the Black and brown disabled stories I remember, I am proud to ground myself in a tradition of, being a grassroots queer of color, disabled intellectual, of working-class history.

1996–2000: *BULLDOZER COMMUNITY NEWS SERVICE*

When I moved to Toronto in 1996/97 as a young, queer femme, brown, Crazy, soon-to-be-disabled twenty-one-year-old, I did it for a lot of reasons: the vibrant queer people of color organizing and cultural scene, the first Sri Lankan community bigger than me and my dad I'd ever lived in, my lover, the fact that I could afford to rent a one-bedroom apartment with a backyard to grow vegetables, the livable wage I could eventually earn once I got papers. But I also came into a community where disability and being a psychiatric survivor and/or abuse survivor were things that were talked about, organized around, not silences in our radical queer and trans Black and brown movements and communities.

One of my first activist commitments was writing for, editing, and distributing *Bulldozer Community News Service,* founded in 1980 and known in earlier incarnations as *Prison News Service. Bulldozer Community News Service* was a radical newspaper that defined its constituencies as prisoners and former prisoners, psychiatric

---

20   Mia Mingus, "About," *Leaving Evidence*, https://leavingevidence.wordpress.com/about-2/, accessed July 16, 2018.

survivors, First Nations[21] people, people of color, and poor people. It was named after the paper's motto: "The only vehicle for prison reform is a bulldozer!"

As *Prison News Service,* the paper had been one of the most important North American prison justice papers in the 1980s and '90s and had developed a strong analysis linking group homes, psychiatric institutions, and prisons as part of the same system—years before radical academics would use the term "carceral systems." White, disabled queer writer Eli Clare would ask in his 2000 book, *Exile and Pride*[22]: What would have happened if the disability and prison justice movements had built alliances in the 1980s, recognizing that prisons and psych institutions and hospitals and nursing homes all lock away people the WSCCAP[23] wants contained? Well, in Toronto, some people were asking that question and organizing around it in 1996. *Bulldozer's* collective was a super working-class, racially mixed collective of young queer people of color, older white working-class ex-prisoners, sex workers, current or former drug users, and survivors of abuse and psychiatrization—most of us were all of the above. Although we might not have seen ourselves as a disability group, disability, PTSD, and madness were deeply interwoven into the social justice journalism

---

21 Throughout this book, I use First Nations (in the way I first heard it in the '90s, and in the way I still hear it used in certain communities in the US, where it was and is used by militant Indigenous writers, activists, and people I knew to assert that their nationhood on Turtle Island was still here and had primacy over white settler colonialists' claims to land and sovereignty). Indigenous and Native refer to Indigenous North American people. I do this not because I think the words all mean the same thing but out of respect for the complex relationships people have with the words we call ourselves, particularly words in colonial languages that have been forced on us, and the ways I have heard many different Native comrades, friends, and people use different terms at different times, fluidly.

22 Eli Clare, "A Challenge to Single-Issue Politics: Reflections from a Decade Later," *Exile and Pride* (Cambridge, MA: South End Press), 1999.

23 The white supremacist capitalist colonialist ableist patriarchy—a delightful term for All That Is Evil, coined by myself, Chanelle Gallant, Arti Mehta, and Loree Erickson around 2010.

we did. We talked and wrote about our experiences as survivors of childhood sexual abuse, PTSD, and madness. Jim Campbell[24], the main editor and longest-standing collective member (who funded *Bulldozer/PNS* almost solely on his wages as a city meter reader), was particularly brave and tone-setting in talking about recovering his memories of being sexually abused as a child in his white, working-class farming community in Northern Ontario, and connections he drew between childhood sexual abuse and colonization, oppression, and prisons. Issues of *Bulldozer* from 1997 contained unsigned (because we wanted to evade surveillance by police and other security institutions like CSIS) articles about how to survive going crazy in jail through books, meditation, and herbs; sex worker organizing against NIMBY (not in my backyard)–style restrictions trying to move street based workers out of the areas where they worked, Mohawk organizer Dacajawaea's recent tour to Toronto, and youth of color breaking out of a new boot camp–style youth jail.

1990S: PSYCH SURVIVOR PRIDE DAY AS A SPACE OF CRAZY, FEMME OF COLOR LEADERSHIP

In the 1980s and '90s, Parkdale, a now heavily gentrified neighborhood in Toronto, was filled with working-class and poor Black and brown people, and known as "Canada's biggest psychiatric ghetto." With the development of long-lasting injectable and pill-based psycho-pharmaceuticals in the 1960s and '70s, 999 Queen West, a.k.a. Queen Street Mental Health, had moved from locking up all its inmates to releasing them into group homes in the community, where you would get a daily allowance of your ODSP or welfare doled out and your

---

24   For more information about Jim, an obituary is available at https://kersplebedeb.com/posts/jim-campbell-remembered/. It includes a reprint of "Fifteen Years of *Bulldozer* and More: The Personal, the Political, and a Few of the Connections, from I 1995" and links to other articles about Jim and *PNS*.

meds monitored. Presented as a humanitarian effort, it was also a profit-maximizing one—it was cheaper to farm out the nuts to group homes than to keep us locked up.

But deinstitutionalization also allowed Crazy people to get together, move more freely, organize about our conditions, and talk about whether we were actually crazy the way the psych system had said we were, or whether maybe we were kinda, but we had also survived abuse, residential school, colonization, and migration.

Psychiatric Survivor Pride Day was one of the places Crazy people got together to organize in Toronto in the 1990s. Founded in 1993 by Lilith Finkler, a queer, working-class Libyan Jewish psych survivor and Parkdale Community Legal Services psychiatric survivor community legal worker—a rare position, someone nuts who had a job helping other Crazy people navigate the system.[25] To me and people I knew, Parkdale Legal was the free social justice legal clinic, a lifeline so many in Parkdale depended on for help with immigration, the legal system, the psych system, or all three. One of the only legal clinics in Canada with a specific focus on mental health law, Parkdale Legal was also a hot spot of poor, people of color, and Crazy community—you ran into everyone there trying to see a worker. Their community legal workers both provided free legal services to poor folks and did community organizing as part of their paid work. (Imagine that.)

As one of those community legal workers, Lilith was a tireless working-class, queer, crazy, femme organizer of color. She taught me so damn much. One of my strongest memories of Lilith is her hanging out and organizing at the Country Site Café, a doughnut shop opposite the Gladstone Hotel. The Gladstone, now a fancy boutique hotel, was then a

25   For an academic article about Psychiatric Survivor Day, see Lilith Finkler, "Psychiatric Survivor Pride Day: Community Organizing with Psychiatric Survivors," *Osgoode Hall Law Journal*, 35, nos. 3–4 (Fall/Winter 1997), Special Issue on Parkdale Community Legal Services: 763–72, https://digitalcommons.osgoode.yorku.ca/cgi/viewcontent.cgi?article=1596&context=ohlj.

pay-by-the-week, down-at-the-heels, gorgeous place where many poor people had lived and built communities for decades. Lots of people who lived at the hotel or in boarding houses or microbachelor apartments in the neighborhood hung out in the doughnut shop all day—it was also a popular place to stop and take a break if you were walking back to the neighborhood from Queen Street Mental Health. Lilith didn't try to organize psych survivors by faxing flyers to social service agencies. Nope—she would hang out at the entrance of Country Site, greet every person in the doughnut shop by name, ask them how they were doing, hand them a flyer for Psych Survivor Pride Day Organizing Committee's meetings, and sometimes offer free legal advice in a corner of the coffee shop. Watching her, it was clear how much she loved other Crazy people and how committed she was to not only leaving no one behind but to making sure that people who had been told they were too nuts to make decisions about anything could make sophisticated political decisions about what action to take. Watching her taught me so damn much.

I went to those meetings as a Crazy, broke, barely-making-it twenty-two- and twenty-three-year-old queer brown femme who was living on about eleven bucks a week for food. I walked three miles each way to the meetings, at a time in my life when my fibromyalgia and chronic fatigue and pain were probably the worst they've ever been—until a horrified Lilith found out and gave me a month's worth of tokens—not the begrudging two that many programs gave out but a whole roll. Those tokens saved my life, and I think Lilith knew and also made absolutely no big deal about it. Those meetings were some of the first meetings where I ran into what I and others would name hallmarks of disability justice culture: free food—that people liked and got to choose—free transit tokens, a physically accessible space, organizing happening at the pace and from the needs of the people doing the organizing, and the belief that Crazy people were not only capable of doing organizing, but that any organizing around psychiatric survivor issues that meant anything had to come from our needs, argument, and desires—not us as window dressing, with the "outcomes" already decided and imposed on us from above like so many social service "community engagement" projects turned out to be. Organizing Psych Survivor Pride Day happened crip styles—slow, starting late, with breaks when someone lost their shit or needed to throw up or cried. We yelled at each other, got triggered, and disagreed. We were "visibly crazy." And we ran things.

And while like in much psych survivor organizing, there were white, cis, straight Crazy dudes who sometimes tried to dominate, in my memory the majority of the participants were Black, brown, and Native women, many of whom were queer. We were led by Lilith, who was great at telling a white Crazy dude to stop yelling at a brown Crazy woman. It was from her queer brown craziness that the idea of a Psychiatric Survivor Pride Day had come—queer people had come up with the idea of Pride, not shame, she said, and psych survivors often both were queer and had a lot of shame to overcome.

The years I was a part of Psych Survivor Pride Day, the stuff we organized included a daylong conference with an opening ceremony by Vern Harper, a Cree Elder who came to many protests and events in Toronto for decades; know-your-rights workshops (about dealing with housing, jobs, dealing with welfare, and the psych system and forced treatment) and healing spaces; a delicious free lunch we got the Catholic Workers to donate that everyone tried to take home; and, best of all, an unpermitted march down the middle of Queen Street. I remember a whole bunch of crazies, including many QT/POC, holding signs and balloons that said, *NO FORCED TREATMENT* and *PROUD TO BE CRAZY*, marching to a boarding house that had recently caught on fire and killed six psych survivors. The impact of seeing a bunch of nuts being a people, marching with dignity and resistance to mourn our dead, assert our humanity, and demand our right to be Crazy without punishment, had a huge impact on both those marching and those watching from the sidewalks.

Lilith left her job in the late 1990s to move to the East Coast and do academic work in disability studies and Madness, and Peggy-Gail Dehal-Ramson, a queer femme Indo-Caribbean organizer, took her place. She changed the name of Psych Survivor Pride Day to Mad Pride, continuing the tradition of Toronto psych survivor organizing led by queer women of color.

1997: EDMOND YU MURDERED BY TORONTO POLICE

Edmond Wai-Hong Yu was a Chinese immigrant who was also a psychiatric survivor. An immigrant from Hong Kong who came to Toronto to attend medical school, he became homeless after a mental health crisis resulted in a paranoid schizophrenia diagnosis and him being forced out of university. On February 20, 1997, normative white people on the Spadina streetcar complained that he was "acting abnormally." Someone called the police. When cops confronted Yu at the back of the streetcar, he pulled out a small hammer he used to crack nuts, and Toronto cop Lou Pasquino shot Yu three times at point-blank range, killing him.[26] Yu was thirty-five when he was murdered.

I had been in Toronto for two weeks, and I remember how it felt to be there then. I remember being a newcomer to the city and to Canada, someone involved in prison justice and anti–police brutality organizing, watching as organizers came together quickly to protest his death. I also noticed how, unlike what I'd witnessed in police brutality organizing in New York, organizers named his murder as both racist and ableist—he was murdered by police because of the interlocking oppressions he faced as a Crazy, houseless, Asian immigrant

---

26   "Letters to the Editor: Bowie but No Glenn Frey?" *Now*, January 27, 2016, https://nowtoronto.com/news/letters-to-the-editor/letters-to-the-editor-bowie-but-no-glenn-frey/, accessed July 16, 2018.

man. Toronto disabled, Crazy, and/or POC organizations, like the Toronto Coalition Against Racism, or TCAR[27] (founded in 1993 after the near-fatal attack of by group of white supremacist skinheads on Sivarajah Vinasithamby, a Sri Lankan Tamil refugee and restaurant worker). I remember my friends pointing out to me and my definitely noticing, how many hot-as-fuck women of color, Black, and First Nations women organizers were in leadership at TCAR. Then there were groups like World Majority Lesbians, the Black Action Defence Committee, the Ontario Coalition Against Poverty, and, yes, Psych Survivor Pride Day.

As a twenty-two-year-old activist, both seasoned at various kinds of activism since I was sixteen and semi-brand new, I both noticed and took for granted then how there was this enormous coalition of people involved in the struggles against police brutality, prisons, and psychiatric survivor issues like forced treatment and forced committals who were coming together and naming them as connected. It just seemed to make sense, how people seemed to understand that prisons, police murder, and psychiatrization were all marinated in racism and colonialism, and were overlapping versions of the same thing—systems to lock us up and kill us. I remember the huge protest march from Yu's murder site at Spadina and King to Queen's Park, thousands of people filling the streets without a permit. It didn't seem odd that people would be able to name racism and Crazy oppression out loud in the same sentence. We were, in some ways, doing disability justice a decade before the invention of the term.

Two decades since that protest, Yu is by far not the last psychiatrized Black or brown person to be murdered by police. In Toronto, Yu's name is on a long list of crazy people who have been shot dead—Otto

---

27   For more on TCAR's history, see Raghu Krishnan "Remembering Anti-Racism," *THIS*, January 1, 2003, https://this.org/2003/01/01/remembering-anti-racism/, accessed July 16, 2018.

Vas, Andrew Loku, Reyal Jardine-Douglas. In Seattle, where I live as I write this, in 2017 multiple Black and Indigenous women labeled "mentally ill" were murdered by police—Charleena Lyles, a pregnant Black mother of five, was shot by police as she held a small knife, when she had called them because she thought someone was breaking into her house. Renee Davis, a member of the Muckleshoot Nation, also a pregnant single mother, was shot by police during a "wellness check." There are official statistics now that show that at least half of the racialized people murdered by law enforcement are also physically or mentally disabled, Deaf, and/or autistic.

There are both protests where we name racism and ableism, and protests where the role ableism plays in our people's deaths gets forgotten. At this moment in time, I remember that we are not the first to remember these connections, know why our people were murdered, and fight like hell to end this world that wants us dead.

2012: SINS INVALID COMES TO TORONTO, SOME SDQTBIPOC TALK

Since Sins Invalid's founding in 2006, our full-scale performances have all occurred in the Bay Area, because the cost to accessibly transport twelve disabled performers and many staff to another part of North America is usually prohibitive. However, beginning in 2010, we began to offer reduced versions of our shows—two to four performers, plus video—to college campuses and venues throughout North America. We usually offered a performance plus a disability justice workshop, viewing both as an organizing opportunity to share our vision of disability justice—centering people of color and queer and trans folks and everyone usually marginalized in mainstream white disability organizing.

In 2011, Sins was approached by Syrus Marcus Ware, a queer, Black, disabled trans artist, cultural worker, co-organizer of Blockorama and Toronto's Prisoners' Justice Film Festival, and youth arts worker at the Art Gallery of Ontario. Ware wanted to bring Sins to Toronto to perform at the AGO. Knowing Ware's groundbreaking work in Black disabled queer/trans culture, I was very excited that SDQTPOC and QTBIPOC communities in Toronto would be able to see a Sins show, live, for free, in a beautiful, accessible theater.

The organizing process was not without challenges, primarily from the racism of the rest of the organizing committee. Ware went on parental leave, which meant that four out of five of the disability studies academics who organized to bring Sins were white disabled people with a history of being racist to disabled Black and brown folks in their disability studies programs. They showed their racism in many ways while we planned the show together by: a) claiming they didn't know any disabled QTBIPOC (despite having kicked SDQTBIPOC out of their academic program or harassed them into leaving); b) asking Loree Erickson, a Toronto-based white, queer, disabled, femme artist, porn creator, and activist with decent anti-racist politics also on the committee, "You seem to know some disabled people of color—can you invite them to join?"; c) saying to a Sins performer (me) during our disability justice workshop, "We're aware we had a diversity problem—that's why we invited you!"; and finally, d) choosing to hold the after-party in bar that, though physically accessible, was a white frat bar adjacent to U of T during Saint Patrick's Day filled with drunk, white, straight, able-bodied patrons and thus *inaccessible* to disabled QTBIPOC because we felt uncomfortable and unsafe. As we prepared to start the show, many Sins artists and SDQTBIPOC gazed nervously at the audience. White/non-disabled people made up more of it than we would've liked and many sick and disabled QTBIPOC, living in the immigrant suburbs or outer ring housing, dependent on the unreliable Wheel-Trans, came late to find the venue at capacity. This could have been prevented by creating priority or reserved seating for SDQTBIPOC at the show. These are the ways in which racist ableism plays out in micro and macro ways in organizing and cultural production.

However, it wasn't all bad. Disabled QTBIPOC organized to house Sins artists and pick them up from the airport, hanging out and building connections. Sins artists and Toronto QTBIPOC artists ditched the party and hung out at a sushi restaurant together after the show. SDQTBIPOC came to the workshop and the performance in numbers, saying that it was literally a show they had been waiting years to see. And some SDQTBIPOC artists, namely myself, Syrus Marcus Ware, Eshan Rafi, Arti Mehta, and Nik Red, went out to brunch the Sunday after and, over gluten-free crepes, shared stories of racism within white disability studies and our ideas for what a Toronto version of Sins could look like.

2013: ELISHA LIM AND LOREE ERICKSON START THE "WHY WOULD I COME TO A PARTY IF MY FRIENDS ARE BARRED?" ACTION

Hello everybody! I have so much tenderness for you, my collective queer brain. This proposition comes with big love:

I QUIT GOING TO PARTIES THAT ARE WHEEL-CHAIR INACCESSIBLE!

This is an act of faith that we can host and demand wheelchair accessible entrances. Feel free to join me, and share this event!

PARTY PLANNERS! You are my people and I love you. You hustle, fundraise, labour and sweat in the name of community. This is Sarah Pinder's awesome spreadsheet of wheelchair accessible party venues. Please contribute to it and consider it when you plan your next party.

Elisha Lim

On January 17, 2013, Elisha Lim, a non-disabled, mixed-race, Asian, genderqueer visual artist, did a small, huge thing: they created a Facebook event. It was called "Why Would I Come to a Party if My Friends are Barred?"[28] In it, they made a public commitment to not attend any inaccessible events for one year.

This action emerged out of Lim's long-term friendship with Loree Erickson, white, queer, femme disabled activist. "It was really personal," said Lim. "I realized I'd been lying to Loree for a couple years where she'd be like, 'What are you doing this weekend?' and I'd say, 'I don't know.'"

The truth that Lim wasn't admitting was that they were going to events that Loree would not be able to go to, because they were inaccessible. Lim explained to me, "I couldn't bear to do it anymore. I decided that I wanted to boycott inaccessible parties just on my own. And then I thought, maybe this is an opportunity to make a public statement."

Lim was amazed at the number of people who joined the Facebook event: almost 400 in the first week. People from across North America became aware of the action, and the Facebook page became an accessible hot spot for people to debate, collectively pool, and cocreate new resources. The event page was the first place I saw Toronto's collectively created Google doc listing accessible performance spaces, started by Toronto queer writer Sarah Pinder. The doc's template was picked up by organizers as far away as Texas who wanted to create a similar resource for their communities.

"The best part about [the action] was the conversations and the fights," said Elisha. I remember those fights; they were huge, on- and offline. Lim recounted facing criticism and backlash from some able-bodied

---

28   To view the archived event and all the commentary, visit Elisha Lim, "Why Would I Come to a Party If My Friends Are Barred?" https://www.facebook.com/events/350503528389995/, accessed July 16, 2018.

queer and trans people of color organizers. People got pissed and said that QTBIPOC event planners without a lot of money were throwing shows in house party or other spaces that were inaccessible but all they could afford. Lim and other organizers responded that most disabled people are poor too. People collectively researched and shared info about affordable, accessible performance spaces, including that you could rent a ramp for thirty-five dollars in Toronto from Shoppers Drug Mart. The Facebook page for the event became an action—a place where disabled QTBIPOC, non-disabled QTBIPOC, and white sick and disabled queers came together to argue and debate and learn. It was a place

People shared and talked about concrete, crip-made accessibility tools like Billie Rain's fragrance-free event resources,[29] the Vancouver white-queer-crip–made blog *Building Radical Accessible Communities Everywhere*[30] and its access audits and posts full of access hacks, like "So if the bathroom in a space you throw events in isn't wheelchair accessible, what are you going to do?" (take the hinges off the door and hang a curtain; rent an accessible porta potty, see if there's a Tim Hortons or other local space nearby with an accessible bathroom and talk to the manager to make sure people can use it) as well as Toronto disability rights organization DAMN 2025's document "How to Book ASL-English Interpreters: An Introduction for (Broke) Community Organizers." Basically, the event page was one big hot spot where people

29   This document can be found at https://dualpowerproductions.com/2011/03/14/ multiple-chemical-sensitivities-mcs-accessibility-basics.

30   "So If the Bathroom in a Space You Throw Events in Isn't Wheelchair Accessible, What Are You Going to Do?", *Radical Accessible Communities*, April 14, 2013, https:// radicalaccessiblecommunities.wordpress.com/2013/04/14/so-if-the-bathroom-in-a-space-you-throw-events-in-isnt-wheelchair-accessible-what-are-you-going-to-do/, accessed July 16, 2018; "Needs and Strategies," *Kindred Healing Justice*, http://www.kindredhealingjustice. org/needs_strategies.html, accessed July 16, 2018; Tanuja Jagernauth, "Jagernauth: Just Healing," *Organizing Upgrade*, October 31, 2010, http://archive.organizingupgrade.com/ index.php/modules-menu/community-care/item/91-jagernauth-just-healing, accessed July 16, 2018.

were drawing on and learning from the already-banked brilliance of low-income sick and disabled folks to create the access we need.

Elisha told me, "People fought a lot, and people really stood their grounds. I feel like it became more trendy to ask, 'Is this party accessible?' Certain parties, like QPOC [a Toronto queer people dance party] moved to accessible spaces because of the action. [S]paces that maybe weren't as 'cool' became cooler because they were accessible. There was a cultural shift." Loree agreed but also noted that many people signed on to the call for solidarity in the Facebook event, but few joined Lim in boycotting every inaccessible party. Both Loree and Elisha felt that the action was a way to use Elisha's able-bodied privilege and cultural capital as a popular non-disabled QTBIPOC artist to raise the profile of accessibility, instead of disabled people always being left with the role of challenging organizers about access and ableism.

I agree. I saw this action and the resources it created as touching off a cultural shift in Toronto, where, for a while in the early 2010s, QTBIPOC performances—even those that weren't specifically disabled or led by disabled folks—began to provide detailed access info; be held at accessible venues like the Tranzac, Gladstone, or Unit 2; and provide ASL or be prepared to face community anger when they failed to. There were community consequences for not being accessible; it was no longer business as usual for able-bodied QTBIPOC organizers to "forget" about accessibility.

Elisha officially ended the Facebook event a year after it began, but the event page is still up, an archive of that electric time. "I feel great because I don't lie to Loree anymore," Elisha said. "To this day I don't go to inaccessible parties, which means I often don't go out at all. Sometimes I feel out of touch and lonely. But people with disabilities feel that way all the time."

2013–15: CRIP YOUR WORLD/PDA: PERFORMANCE/DISABILITY/ART

Remember that gluten-free brunch after the Sins AGO performance? It didn't stop there. Through emails and texts, many failed and one successful grant application, me and Syrus Ware hatched a plan to launch a Toronto-based, QTBIPOC-majority disability art collective: Performance/Disability/Art (PDA). Our QTBIPOC show *Crip Your World: An Intergalactic 2QT/POC Sick and Disabled Extravaganza* brought together ten sick, disabled, Deaf, and Mad video and live disability justice performance artists from North America for a sold-out show at the 2014 Mayworks Festival. Later that year, we planned and carried out a cross-disabled, QT/POC–centered arts retreat called The Great Disability Arts Retreat. The workshops lasted eight weeks. We'd meet and hang out and talk about our work and what it means to be a crip writer or artist not only in a world that has so many invisible and ableist barriers but also a world that assumes we're not be able to create at all ... Our latest show, *PDA Takes Over the Artists' Newsstand*, was a case in point—when we were invited to perform in an inaccessible venue (a takeover of an unused newsstand in the inaccessible Chester subway station), we highlighted its inaccessibility by creating a crip arts march from Broadview, the closest accessible subway station, and by filling the subway station with disabled art, ASL interpretation, many people sitting and taking up space with our scooters, wheelchairs, canes, pain, signing, and Madness.

We continue to meet, create, and perform on a crip basis—"as spoons allow," as cocreator Syrus Marcus Ware says. I believe our small, important space has helped other sick and disabled arts spaces populated by QTBIPOC grow. I would like to believe our work makes other SDQTBIPOC artists feel like they can throw a big show, write a big complicated work. Writing about our arts practice makes me think about many questions about disability justice arts practice. What does it mean to make disabled art space that is richly Black and brown, poor, cross-abled, with childcare, cheap, and moving at the slow, sick, canceling, Access-A-Ride-broke-down pace of our bodies? Often, it means not producing at the "hot shot," "ambitious" able-bodied pace of abled arts practice, even abled QTBIPOC practice. Are we seen as less serious because of that? How can we keep insisting on our slow-moving, strong, and vulnerable SDQTBIPOC arts practice?

This chapter is still being written.

SICK AND CRAZY HEALER

A NOT-SO-BRIEF PERSONAL HISTORY OF THE HEALING JUSTICE MOVEMENT

> *Our movements themselves have to be healing, or there's no point to them.*
> —Cara Page, Kindred Southern Healing Justice Collective

PRO TIPS/POP QUIZ:

Those words: "Sick." "Disabled." "Healer." Do you think of them in the same sentence?

Do you think a sick, mad, Deaf, neurodivergent, and/or disabled person can heal?

What do you think "healing" is? Do you think that it means becoming as close to able-bodied as possible?

Do you think it is always sad or terrible to be sick or disabled? Do you think everybody wants to be able-bodied and neurotypical, and would choose it if they could?

Does healing justice mean to you that someday no one will be disabled or sick because there will be no toxic waste and health care for all?

Everyone I know longs for healing. It's just hard to get. The good kind of healing: healing that is affordable, has childcare and no stairs, doesn't misgender us or disrespect our disabilities or sex work, believes us when we're hurt and listens when we say what we need, understands that we are the first and last authority on our own bodies and minds.

Most folks I know come to activist spaces longing to heal, but our movements are often filled with more ableism and burnout than they are with healing. We work and work and work from a place of crisis. Healing is dismissed as irrelevant, reserved for folks with money, an individual responsibility, something you do on your own time. Our movements are so burnout-paced, with little to no room for grief, anger, trauma, spirituality, disability, aging, parenting, or sickness, that many people leave them when we age, have kids, get sick(er) or more disabled, or just can't make it to twelve meetings a week anymore.

A HEALING LINEAGE

I've been involved in what's known as the healing justice movement since 2010, and have been involved and invested in healing as a form of liberation and social justice all my life—from when I was a little survivor brown femme disabled kid to when I was a nineteen-year-old feeling ashamed of her altar and interest in herbs and tarot because they were a "departure from the real struggle." The healing justice movement was created in response to all of those things— from burnout to ableist movement cultures that denigrate and dismiss healing as not serious, to a lack of access to high-quality healing and health care by oppressed people—and in the hope of reclaiming the ways our oppressed, surviving communities have always healed, from before colonization to now.

Healing justice as a movement and a term was created by queer and trans Black, Indigenous, and People of color, beginning with the work of Kindred Southern Healing Justice Collective in 2004, to define a movement of politicized Black and brown healers reclaiming our traditional methods of healing and redefine what healing and health could mean, especially in terms of dealing with intergenerational trauma.

Of course before "healing justice" was a term, healers had been healing folks at kitchen tables and community clinics for a long time—from the acupuncture clinics run by Black Panthers like Mutulu Shakur in North America in the 1970s to our bone-deep Black, Indigenous, people of color and pre-christian European traditions of healing with herbs, acupuncture, touch, prayer, and surgery. As my mentor, intuitive healer Dori Midnight, says, "It's nothing new to invite people into your home, give them some tea, listen to their grief, hold space for their pain, lay them down on cushions on the floor and pray with them or touch them or move energy and offer them remedies made from plants and stones."

The healing justice practice spaces (HJPSs) I've been at—at big conferences and small ones, in corners of protests and small community spaces like Third Root and Harriet's Apothecary, and in actions like Healing Justice for Black Lives Matter—have felt like a temple and a balm. In Detroit, at the 2010 USSF, the HJPS was in an old union hall. There was an altar in the entranceway holding a bowl filled with Detroit water and other waters healers had brought from all over the continent and beyond. People sat quietly in a circle as they received community acupuncture. The schedule of healers was scrawled on sheets of big paper in Magic Marker: Reiki, somatics, herbs, community acupuncture, counseling, tarot. People who were scared of the doctor's office could come there, breaking their isolation and shame about needing care. We were creating a movement that could be care-full. I have seen healing justice practice spaces as the temple, the balm in the middle of movement hecticness. Places where healing shifts the ways we imagine movement organizing to be.

One of the guiding forces who helped birth healing justice is Cara Page. A Black and Indigenous Southern queer femme organizer and heart, Page's work with the Kindred Southern Healing Justice Collective and the Healing Justice People's Movement Assembly at the 2010 Detroit United States Social Forum were foundational for what would become healing justice. Kindred, a collective of queer Black and brown Southern healers, came to be in 2007, when they noticed that Black and brown Southern organizers, particularly those working in New Orleans in the wake of Hurricane Katrina, were literally dying from stress, exhaustion, and trauma.[31] In their "Needs and Strategies" statement, the collective asserts, "We need to be able to respond to the increased state of burnout and depression in our movements; systematic loss of our communities' healing traditions; the isolation and stigmatization of healers; and the increased privatization of our land, medicine and natural resources that has caused us to rely on state or private models we do not trust and that do not serve us."[32]

One of the first collectives to talk about the importance of healing within a movement, not as a sidenote but as a core practice, Kindred took those visions to meet with other radical healers at the 2010 Detroit US Social Forum to create perhaps the first ever politicized healers' gathering at a giant leftist North American gathering tasked with visioning the future. At the 2010 USSF Healing Justice People's Movement Assembly, one of many large scale gatherings on topics to occur at the USSF to draft resolutions and visionary future plans, I heard Cara say something that has stuck with me ever since: "Our movements themselves need to be healing, or there is no point to them." This shook me. The idea that movements themselves could and should be spaces of healing, that care didn't have to be a sideline to "the real work" but could *be* the work, was like a deep drink of clear water. It was something I'd been longing for for years. I think healing justice is a space of longing. I took that water

31   For more about Kindred, see *Healing Collective Trauma*'s collection of interviews with the collective at http://www.healingcollectivetrauma.com/kindred-collective-wellness-within-liberation .html and Prentis Hemphill, "Healing Justice Is How We Can Sustain Black Lives," *Huffington Post*, https://www.huffingtonpost.com/entry/healing-justice_us_5899e8ade4b0c1284f282ffe, accessed July 16, 2018.

32   *Kindred Southern Healing Justice Collective*, http://kindredhealingjustice.org/, accessed May 9, 2016.

and that knowledge back with me from Detroit, quietly determined that I would figure out a way to find the places where the movement work healed us, instead of burning us out. And if I couldn't find them, I would help make some.

SICK AND CRAZY HEALER: ONE WAY THIS CAN LOOK

I am a disabled and chronically ill healer. I am a survivor of childhood sexual abuse who has complex PTSD and the trigger land mines, who swims in the anxiety and panic oceans, for whom pills were not a safe or accessible option, so I started growing motherwort in my backyard and making tinctures out of cheap vodka. I am a nonbinary femme of Irish, Romany, Burgher, and Tamil Sri Lankan ascent who started reading cards as a deeply depressed nineteen-year-old whose mom was then dying of cancer and first femme girlfriend was suicidal. I am that femme who read tarot for phone-about-to-be-cut-off money, at the queer dance party, on a psychic hotline when my part-time rape crisis line contract ended. I am the activist who has had an altar since I can remember but only came out of the (broom) closet about how deeply spiritual I was as the QTBIPOC witch revolution began to bloom. I am the person who, years later, in Oakland, was drawn to the healing justice movement when it started to be a thing, even as I kept questioning whether I was "really a healer."

Six years ago, when I had zero dollars in my bank account and rent was due, I created and posted up an "I can read your tarot cards" WordPress site and was bowled over by the response. As I launched my tarot business in a more intentional way, one rooted in the healing justice movement in the Bay Area and beyond, I started breathing in that this could be "real"—that being a community healer, in a "community healer-full movement,"[33] could be a real way of both paying my rent and

---

33   In coining the phrase "healer-full," I am riffing off of Black Lives Matter's Black, queer, feminist conception of BLM as a "leader-full movement," one that eschews a few straight,

playing a role in our communities. I've participated as a co-organizer and healer in healing justice practice spaces at the Allied Media Conference, Communities United Against Violence's Safetyfest,[34] and INCITE!'s Color of Violence 4 conference in Chicago, as well as smaller spaces in collective houses. I helped co-coordinate the AMC's 2013 Healing Justice Network Gathering, which brought together many healers from across North America to talk about ableism, cultural appropriation, and funding our work. With Susan Raffo and Adaku Utah, I helped organize the 2014 Healing Justice for Black Lives Matter fundraiser, where healing justice practitioners came together across North America to raise money for the Ferguson bail fund through healing en masse on the winter solstice.

IF IT'S NOT ANTI-ABLEIST, IT'S NOT HEALING JUSTICE

> We center the genius and leadership of disabled and chronically ill communities, for what we know about surviving and resisting the medical industrial complex and living with fierce beauty in our sick and disabled bodies. We say no to the medical industrial complex's model of "cure or be useless," instead working from a place of belief in the wholeness of disability, interdependence and disabled people as inherently good as we are.
> —from the 2012 Allied Media Conference Healing Justice Practice Space Guiding Principles

---

cis, male, able-bodied leaders but is also not "leaderless"—where many people, especially femme, female, trans, disabled, and poor/working-class/rural people who have had our work erased get to be recognized as leaders and organizers.

34 Safetyfest was a late great festival held from 2010 to 2012 by Communities United Against Violence (CUAV), a Bay Area queer and trans anti-violence organization. Safetyfest was the most mammoth QT mostly BIPOC festival ever, throwing something like seventeen workshops and events in twelve days with the aim of making anti-violence work in queer and trans communities sexy, fun, and liberatory.

I am a chronically ill and crazy intuitive healer, and I cancel a lot. I've canceled a lot in my sick and disabled life, and I will continue to cancel—whether it's because I start puking or have a panic attack or my hips hurt so bad I can't think—until I am dead.

I cancel on parties and appointments and life, but I also cancel on my clients. I heal with this brilliant sick and disabled bodymind. This may sound cute, and trust me, it often is, but it also means constant pleasurable and stressful labor to undo, oh, I don't know, the entire impact of ableism and the settler colonial medical-industrial complex on how we think about what healing is.

Mainstream ideas of "healing" deeply believe in ableist ideas that you're either sick or well, fixed or broken, and that nobody would want to be in a disabled or sick or mad bodymind. Unsurprisingly and unfortunately, these ableist ideas often carry over into healing spaces that call themselves "alternative" or "liberatory." The healing may be acupuncture and herbs, not pills and surgery, but assumptions in both places abound that disabled and sick folks are sad people longing to be "normal," that cure is always the goal, and that disabled people are objects who have no knowledge of our bodies. And deep in both the medical-industrial complex and "alternative" forms of healing that have not confronted their ableism is the idea that disabled people can't be healers.

Most sick and disabled people I know approach healing wanting specific things—less pain, less anxiety, more flexibility—but not usually to become able-bodied. And many of us don't feel automatically comfortable going to healing spaces at all because of our histories of being seen as freaks, scrutinized, infantilized, patronized with "What happened?" prayed over, and asked, "Have you tried acupuncture?" and a million other "miracle cures." Able-bodied practitioners without an anti-ableist analysis—including Reiki providers and anti-oppression therapists—often see us as objects of disgust, fascination, and/or inspiration porn. Mostly, these practitioners dismiss our lived expertise about our bodyminds and their needs, or on the flip side, they tell us we're "not really disabled!" when we insist on the realities of our lives. This carries over into organizing, where, even in HJ spaces, often when the crips aren't there, there's no access info and no accessibility.

I believe healing justice must centralize anti-ableism as a central tenet of the work we do, centering crip ideas of what illness and disability are, as well as honoring disabled and sick and mad people's autonomy and wisdom, and centralizing accessibility in a broad sense (from wheelchair access to fragrance access to ASL presence) as a central part of how we heal, not an add-on or an afterthought. Many of the BIPOC who were first involved in early HJ initiatives were themselves disabled or were close comrades with people birthing early disability justice ideas circa 2010. As the movement grows, I see more HJ spaces up a flight or two of stairs, including ones run by people in my communities, where practitioners seem surprised when crips show up or are angry at lack of access.

Access doesn't just happen—anywhere—and there are specific challenges and tasks to making a healing space accessible. In screening healers who applied to practice at an HJPS, we've had to ask specific questions about the practitioners' understandings of disability, ableism, and healing, as well as fatness; educate people on language and access 101; figure out if the space we were offered was really accessible or the staff were just saying that; and work with healers to make their practices fragrance-free. Most healers or medical care providers never receive any education about the medical-industrial complex, disabled people, or ableism as part of their training. We remake ideas of healing away from being fixed and towards being autonomously and beautifully imperfect.

WHERE WE ARE NOW: A MOVEMENT AT MIDLIFE

In 2018, eight years after I first encountered the language of healing justice, it feels to me that we're at the time in movements where some of the people, moments, articles, wishes that birthed us are at risk of being forgotten—especially in low-money, low-time-to-document, brilliant-burn-out-femme-of-color–led movements. It could be the moment when disability gets forgotten, when class gets forgotten, when white, cis, able-bodied healers can try to slap "healing justice" on their spaces and try to forget that this movement was birthed by Black and brown disabled femme brilliance, in response to all that both mainstream Western/biomedical and "alternative" white/cis/abled spaces lack in terms of understanding how colonialism, ableism, cultural theft, and whorephobia affect healing systems. In response, I offer some of these memories and moments, reflections and recipes of why we do this, what healing justice is to me, and where we might go from here.

So eight years in, what are some thoughts I have about the state of the movement, on what we are doing, and what I think is important to remember?

If an HJ space is all or mostly white queers, it's no different from any "mainstream alternative" white space. Healing justice was created as a term and a movement in part because a lot of "alternative healing" was dominated by white middle- to upper-middle-class people doing culturally appropriative work with nary an analysis of race and a high fee for service. But fast-forward to late 2014, when we did the Healing Justice for Black Lives Matter action. At first, this was a majority BIPOC action, but a million white people started to jump in to "help," and everything started to change. We had to ask that everyone who participated have information about the origins of Black Lives Matter—that it was created by three Black women, two of whom are queer—and think about access, from both a disability and a BIPOC framework, offering, for example, free treatments for Black organizers and community members affected by grief over Black death.

If white healers slap "healing justice" on their work but are still using the healing traditions of some folks' cultures that aren't their own, are primarily working and treating white middle-class

and upper-class people, are unaware or don't recognize that HJ was created by Black and brown femmes, are not working with a critical stance and understanding of how colonization, racism, and ableism are healing issues ... it ain't healing justice. I'm not here for HJ becoming just a white people thing. And neither is HJ.

Who Is a Real Healer? We all are/can be. When I started participating in HJ, like almost every healer I know, I asked myself, *What am I doing? I'm not really a healer.* Every healer from oppressed communities I have ever met has had similar thoughts. Many of our traditional BIPOC forms of healing were outlawed by enslavement and settler colonialism, and then stolen by white people who take our healing traditions, apply certification programs that exclude many of us, and sell them for a profit. So, many of us can't financially afford to learn our own traditions and/or stomach the racism in the existing trainings and have impostor syndrome. But—fuck that.

It's also a revolution to reclaim what it looks like to be a crip healer, a parenting healer, a sex-working healer, a poor/working-class healer. Healing can happen in corners of rooms or on Skype, can start late, can cancel because of a flare. Can be sick, weird, curse, happen in a corner of the BLM encampment in a drizzle. Can be a haircut, a blow job, an accessible dance party, a Reiki treatment—or all four at once.

A little money would help. We do a lot on a little, but we need to figure out how to support each other and resource each other so these big healing dreams can keep growing instead of crashing and burning. Every movement has an initial growth spurt where we can go a long way on joy and adrenaline, but that initial booster rocket doesn't last forever. Maryse Mitchell-Brody, therapist, organizer, and cofounder of Rock Dove Collective, a healing justice collective that operated from 2006 to 2014 in New York, remarked, "A lot of those little HJ collectives that started around 2010 and faded around 2015 would've lasted longer with even small stipends for all the free work we put in."

This is an especially important point when we consider that most of the HJ collectives and spaces I know of were created and are sustained by working-class Black and brown femme labor—femme labor that is often not valued or seen as work. In my years living in Oakland, I estimate that I worked for ten hours a week on unpaid healing justice organizing; my paid practice usually took another ten to twenty hours a week with unpaid time to buy supplies, do rituals, and get support. It took 'til I moved back to Toronto in 2014 and stopped participating in Bay Area healing justice organizing for me to realize how many unpaid hours of work I was doing a week, and how both nurturing and exhausting they were. As we keep going, can we share skills about how to get paid for organizing and healing, how we can share money and create cross-class solidarity?

It doesn't have to be either healing or organizing: it's both. Someone asked me at a talk I was giving at Portland State University's Take Back the Night how we choose between healing and activism. I tried to tell them that healing justice is not a spa vacation where we recover from organizing and then throw ourselves back into the grind. To me, it means a fundamental—and anti-ableist—shift in how we think of movement organizing work to think of it as a place where building in many pauses, where building in healing, where building in space for grief and trauma to be held makes the movements more flexible and longer lasting.

Grief is an important part of the work. So many of the movements I've been a part of in my lifetime—the movements against wars in Afghanistan/Iraq and against Islamophobic racist violence here on Turtle Island, movements for sex work justice and for missing and murdered Indigenous women, movements led by and for trans women of color, movements for Black lives, movements by and for disabled folks and for survivors of abuse—involve a lot of grieving and remembering people we love who have been murdered, died, or been hurt/abused/gone through really horrible shit. Yet I remember an older brown activist telling me in 2003 that there was no time for crying over the use of shock and awe during the invasion of Iraq; we had to get into the streets. Although containing and denying grief is a time-honored activist practice that works for some people, I would argue that feelings of grief and trauma are not a distraction from the struggle. For example, transformative justice work—strategies that create justice, healing, and safety for survivors of abuse without predominantly relying on the state—is hard as hell! What would it be like if we built healing justice practices into it from the beginning? Everything from praying to the goddesses of transformation to help us hold these giant processes and help someone acting abusively choose to change to having cleansing ceremonies along the way. I've witnessed and read about Black Lives Matter organizers integrating healing justice practices into BLM organizing and talking about BLM itself as a healing justice movement—one where at the work's center are grief rituals over murdered Black kin, breath work, and herbs for resilience during actions and marches.[35]

It's not about self-care—it's about collective care. Collective care means shifting our organizations to be ones where people feel fine if they get sick, cry, have needs, start late because the bus broke down, move slower, ones where there's food at meetings, people work from home—and these aren't things we apologize for. It is the way we do the work, which centers disabled-femme-of-color ways of being in the world, where many of us have often worked from our sickbeds, our kid beds, or our too-crazy-to-go-out-today beds. Where we actually care for each other and don't leave each other behind. Which is what we started with, right?

---

35   For some examples, see "Emotional + Physical Safety in Protests," https://justhealing. files.wordpress.com/2012/04/emotional-physical-safety-in-protests-blm.pdf; "Practices for Moving through Grief," https://justhealing.files.wordpress.com/2012/04/practices-for-moving-through-grief-blm.pdf; and "Self-Care for Trauma, Grief + Depression," https:// justhealing.files.wordpress.com/2012/04/self-care-for-trauma-grief-and-depression-blm. pdf.

As my friend and comrade queer yoga teacher Yashna Maya Padamsee, a 2010 HJPS co-organizer and writer, wrote in her often cited article "Communities of Care, Organizations for Liberation": "If we let ourselves be caught up in the discussion of self-care we are missing the whole point of Healing Justice (HJ) work ... Too often self-care in our organizational cultures gets translated to our individual responsibility to leave work early, go home—alone—and go take a bath, go to the gym, eat some food and go to sleep. So we do all of that 'self-care' to return to organizational cultures where we reproduce the systems we are trying to break."[36]

THE FUTURE

I remember the Healing Together Network Gathering at the 2013 Allied Media Conference, a "network gathering," or mini-conference, the day before the AMC proper. I was one of six co-coordinators who had worked for almost a year on the gathering. The gathering was a lot of things for me. There were some amazing meetings of the minds, trainings, and connections. For me, it was also a lesson in the difficulties of trying to organize a financially and disability accessible North America–wide conference on a budget of less than $2,000.

In my Taurus organizer head, I'd hoped that a North American network would emerge out of the gathering that would connect the many different healers, healing justice collectives, and microclinics blooming across the continent. It didn't happen. When a friend saw my face fall, she said that one of the principles of emergence theory is that networks and organizing are organic. We need to trust that need and desire and conditions we are alive to will help us create the networks and structures that serve us. What is easy is accessible, and replicable.

Five years later, I have even more questions: What happens to a

---

36 Yashna Maya Padamsee, "Communities of Care, Organizations for Liberation," *Naya Maya*, June 19, 2011, http://nayamaya.wordpress.com/2011/06/19/communities-of-care-organizations-for-liberation/, accessed July 16, 2018.

movement as it becomes popular, as the dusty old resources are lost? I'm a semiretired witch, no longer making half my income and spending half my time reading cards and practicing intuitive counseling with people. Many of the healing justice collective spaces I came up around—SAGE, Rock Dove, Living Room Project—have ceased operating, closed by gentrification of affordable spaces or burnout. When I started, I could name two other tarot readers who were queer people of color; today, there are what feels like a million "Instagram witches." Some of the HJ spaces I know are still up a flight of stairs, and I wonder if anyone really took in what I thought we were all on the same page about disability.

Yet I also hold to the wild truth that as long as we need to heal, we will continue to dream into being the exact kinds of healing we need. I know sick and disabled healers, whatever we call ourselves, will continue to find ways to offer the particular kinds of crooked, cripped-out healing only we can offer. For the simple reason that this is what we have always done. I just want us to keep cripping-out all our movements—including these precious and sacred ones where we create new and old spaces to heal.

2012 ALLIED MEDIA CONFERENCE HEALING JUSTICE PRACTICE SPACE PRINCIPLES AND GUIDELINES

We begin by listening.

We are people of color, indigenous people, disabled people, and survivors of trauma, many genders, ages and classes of people, and we are committed to leading the work of building healing justice at the AMC.

We do this work to lift up and politicize the role of health and healing in our movements as a critical part of the new world we are building.

We honor individual and community agency, intuition, and innate wisdom, and therefore honor people's rights to make decisions about their own bodies.

We understand that health and wellness should be determined by the individual or community receiving care, and for many of us this includes the reality of disability, illness, and harm reduction. We accept and encourage individuals and communities defining health, healing, and wellness for themselves, and not based on normative models of healing.

We center the genius and leadership of disabled and chronically ill communities, for what we know about surviving and resisting the medical industrial complex and living with fierce beauty in our sick and disabled bodies. We say no to the medical industrial complex's model of "cure or be useless," instead working from a place of belief in the wholeness of disability, interdependence and disabled people as inherently good as we are.

We live in countries that deny health care access to people based on economic and identity status, and we must build alternative structures for giving and receiving care that are grounded in community and ancestral traditions and in the values of consent and equality. The Healing Justice Practice Space is a part of that work.

We believe that medicine is media, and we work with the understanding that how we heal ourselves is directly related to how we see and interpret ourselves and the possibility for transformation.

We are aware that the body does not live forever, and that we honor death as a part of the cycle of life.

HEALING & HEALTH JUSTICE COLLECTIVE ORGANIZING PRINCIPLES
US SOCIAL FORUM, DETROIT, JUNE 2010

We are committed to People of Color & Indigenous leadership, in partnership with our allies, on building healing justice work at the USSF.

We will lift up the leadership and conditions of Detroit to define the healing justice practice space and other programming for healing justice inside of a national context.

We enter this work through an anti-oppression framework that seeks to transform and politicize the role of healing inside of our movements and communities.

We are learning and creating this political framework about a legacy of healing and liberation that is meeting a particular moment in history inside of our movements that seeks to: regenerate traditions that have been lost; to mindfully hold contradictions in our practices; and to be conscious of the conditions we are living and working inside of as healers and organizers in our communities and movements.

We are building national relationships and dialogues to cultivate knowledge and to build reflection and exchange of our healing, transformative and resiliency practices in our regions and movements.

We believe in transparency on all levels so that we can have a foundation of trust, openness and honesty in our vision and action together.

We believe in open source knowledge; which means that all information and knowledge is to be shared and transferred to create deeper collaboration and cross-movement building strategy.

As we continue to create spaces for healing and sustainability throughout the US Social Forum and beyond; we will keep ourselves in mind as well as conscious of our own capacity and well being.

We believe in movement building and organizing within an anti-racist and anti-hierarchical framework that builds collective decision making, strategies, vision and action and does not seek to support only one model or one approach over others.

We believe that there is no such thing as joining this process too late; as we move forward, anyone who comes in when they come in are welcomed; and we will always remember that we are interconnected with many communities, struggles and legacies who have joined healing and resiliency practices with liberation in their work for centuries.

CRIP SEX MOMENTS AND THE LUST OF RECOGNITION

A CONVERSATION WITH E.T. RUSSIAN

This piece is a transcription of a conversation between myself and white, disabled, genderqueer visual artist E.T. Russian and was one of several short videos disabled, queer, Korean activist and writer Mia Mingus filmed and placed on her website in the early 2010s. This was very early on in the smartphone/easy digital video era, and we were all amazed that you could buy a tiny camera and shoot tiny videos and upload them and immediately reach hundreds of people. We absolutely were excited about talking about disabled lives, questions, and culture-making and to spread these ideas to the masses, especially the crip masses!

In Mia's words contextualizing the original piece, "Here is the first of many-to-come videos of snap shots of some of the brilliance and deep complexities that we hold individually and collectively, as a people. We must leave evidence ... Recently, I met up with Leah Lakshmi Piepzna-Samarasinha and E.T. Russian for an evening and got to capture some of our musings, sharings and stories. Whenever I get to hear crip stories, I am entranced. I love hearing our words (all of them, in whatever way they come tumbling out) and feel ever-so appreciative, especially knowing how long I went without ever hearing any of our voices tell our own stories and stumble through sharing and asking and loving. It's so important for us to tell our stories—to each other. As much as we can. There are so many different stories that we have to tell about (queer) crip sex and about our relationship to crip sex, to sex period, to sexuality and more. Our stories are so different and complex and they all have value—we have value. Much love and gratitude to Leah and E.T. for sharing some of your stories, knowing that it's not all of your story."

I had first encountered E.T.'s work in the mid-'90s when I read their zine, Ring of Fire, *which focused on their experiences as a new amputee exploring sex, genderqueerness, kink, and disability.* Ring of Fire *was one of the first places people I knew that encountered writing about disability, from a queer and punk perspective. Fifteen years later, we met again when E.T. was doing makeup artistry for Sins Invalid's 2009 show. During a brunch hangout the day after the show, some of us started talking about feedback Black, queer wheelchair dancer Alice Sheppard had written on her blog after seeing the show—that while she appreciated the hotness of the performance, she wanted more than positive portrayals of disabled sexuality. She wanted someone to do a piece about what it was like when your catheter falls out during sex and you spray your partner in the face with urine. E.T. and I became friends and artistic collaborators, and began to write and dream some of those real-life, complicated crip sexuality stories that hover between joy, shame, and just being. Our conversation came out of that time.*

Leah: [Laughing] I don't want to ever have sex with anyone but another chronically ill or disabled person again. I'm just like, oh god, it's such a relief.

HOW DO YOU DEFINE CRIP LUST?

Leah: Loving and having really good sex in a very broadly defined way with another disabled or chronically ill person where you're lusting towards each other in a sexual fashion.

WHAT DO YOU MEAN WHEN YOU USE THE PHRASE "CRIP SEX MOMENTS"?

Leah: The first thing that comes to my mind is when my lover at the time and me were at this queer club night and they threw me up against the wall and we were making out. And then we both lost our balance at the same time and we totally fell over onto the ground onto the ass of my friend who had been hit by a car a year ago, so then she fell over. So, we're all on the floor in this writhing mass of disabled bodies and it was really great. [Laughing]

E.T.: I've had a disability for fourteen years and I've had several long-term relationships. In between I've dated a lot of different kinds of people—some with disabilities, really different disabilities than me. I've never ... well, okay, once I dated someone who was also an amputee.

Crip sex can be no different at all than sex with nondisabled people, and sometimes it can be really, really different. Like, my partner has no feeling from the chest down and there's a catheter and a leg bag with urine in it and that's in the bed with us. Or, I kiss my date in an elevator and, oops, the force of me kissing them knocks them over in their wheelchair. Then they're on the ground and we have to figure out how to transfer them back up in their wheelchair ... Like all that kind of stuff.

And then there are the times where I have a new date who is not disabled ... When they don't know how my legs work and I have to explain how my legs work because my legs come off. Usually that's not a big deal. I've really only dated one person who wasn't comfortable with my disability. She was like, "Oh, hospitals, they just make me feel uncomfortable. I just don't like them." And I was like, "Wow, I've spent a lot of time in hospitals. They're kind of my home away from home, because I've had to spend so much time in them for my own appointments and stuff." So, I was like, "That's cool, I think we're just in a really different place." She also bicycled a lot and would go on these forty-mile bike trips and I just couldn't relate.

Leah: You were really compatible. [Joking]

E.T.: Yeah, we were incompatible. [Laughing]

But on the other hand, I'm dating someone right now who bikes a lot, and we've had really cool conversations about how that whole bicycling culture can be super alienating, and they're awesome about it. Like, they don't care that we drive around a lot in my truck. A lot of people have car guilt. When you have a mobility-related disability, you kinda have to get over the car guilt. So ... we make out in my truck all the time, and I have to say, it's pretty great. [Laughs]

Leah: When I was twenty-six, I'd been celibate for a couple years because I was dealing with being a sexual abuse survivor and I kinda re-broke my virginity with this totally awesome queer man of color who was really perverted, who had severe RSI. Who was this total, like, Black science fiction polyamorous geek porn maker, with injury stuff and whose primary partner had fibromyalgia too. So, not only was I fucking this amazing hot QPOC in leather pants, but I was like, "Oh my hips just went out," and he was like, "Yeah, no problem. Great. Let's just move positions."

And then there's the stuff that's just like the hard stuff we go through, but then also the really weird stuff that we don't get to talk about. Like, what happens when you lose control of your bowels during sex? [Laughing] You know, all kinds of stuff, right? What's it really like?

THE LUST OF RECOGNITION

Leah: I think we were talking about the healing of recognition, or the erotics of recognition?

E.T.: We talked about the lust of recognition.

Leah: The lust of recognition! Yes! I think it's like any identity stuff. I mean, the first time I fucked someone else who was South Asian, I was like—and I mean, I know it's corny to talk about "going home," but I felt that. And there was something really healing about that. And when I was lovers with the lover I mentioned before and I was like, oh I never have to worry about you being freaked out about me needing to take a break because I'm an incest survivor. Or me needing to negotiate my body in different ways. You don't freak out over that because you're really—you've dated a lot of crips, you are a crip, your primary partner has a bunch of chronic illnesses. And you're just like, "Right, yeah, bodies, work it out." And how amazing that was and how that crip knowledge was so tied to that person's awareness around consent, in the middle of being a big pervert who's into a lot of pretty intense SM. I mean, it was amazing. It was really, really, really amazing. I felt so lucky. I was so lucky.

E.T.: I identify a lot with people who use a wheelchair sometimes and can sometimes also walk, because that's my experience. Where not every day looks the same, in terms of how you get around. I relate to that, obviously, because that's what happens for me.

So ... I see this person around, I think they're cute, they have a cane, there's something really hot about that. Then we meet. They're pretty nice and very cute. And then I notice ... their ankle brace, their cane, their missing fingers (or something like that). And I get to know them a little better and realize ... I'm really attracted. I realize I'm attracted to the fact that they're walking with a cane and they're cute. And then, there's this process I go through: *Am I fetishizing their cane?* I've been writing about this on and off the last couple of years. Is it a fetish? Or is it that I recognize myself in the cane? And there's that lust of recognition. There's something really charged for me, where I just crush out. It's hot. I feel drawn—like a magnet—to the person. They have to be an awesome person that's cute in other ways—it's not just the cane [Leah laughing]—but there's something. It's like this extra electric charge that's there for me and it's very real.

I don't need to only date other disabled people, but a lot of those experiences I've had have been really powerful. Even if not always lasting. I need to be fed in so many different ways. Who's to say what the rest of my life will look like, but there's something about that lust of recognition, that connection ... I think it's good to check in with myself, like *am I fetishizing them???*, but I don't really have a lot of guilt or weirdness around that, because I don't necessarily think that I am.

Leah: Yeah, I wouldn't waste your time.

E.T.: Yeah.

THE GOOD, THE BAD, THE UGLY, AND THE REAL

Leah: So when you were like, "What's crip sex, Leah?" And I was like, "Well, I think it's crips lusting for other crips—yes, that." And I think what you were just saying, E.T., makes me think that I think it's any form of sex that involves someone who is disabled. So, like, I've had crip sex that was shitty, like me being a disabled person who was having sex with a partner who didn't get it. One of my long-term partners was white, working class, genderqueer—actually raised rural poor—and we bonded over class, because I grew up working class, lower middle class, a lot as working class. And we both identified as being people who were less than middle class in movements that were very middle class. And, you know, I really got where she was coming from, she was like, "Yeah, you know, we don't admit disability, we just tough it out, because we don't have that option." And I was like, "Totally, yeah. My mom had polio and they didn't have money for health care, so her doctor that she saw—true story—was like, 'Here's a bicycle, ride it out.'" And my mom [E.T. laughing] ... no, seriously.

E.T.: Wow.

Leah: Yeah. And my mom worked two or three jobs the whole time that I knew her, and it was only when I was older that I was like, "Oh she can't really walk far, without being in a lot of pain," but she would never identify as disabled. Anyway, so back to my girlfriend: I got that she was like, "Whatever, we just tough it out. No problem."

I mean, she had worked construction and she'd be like, "Yeah, I got a nail gun through my finger, I just kept going." [Laughing] Yeah, that was a fascinating relationship. You know, the sex that I had with that person was crip sex because I was in it, but it wasn't necessarily crip-accepting sex, and that's what a lot of us have too.

I guess I'm trying to spin something off of what you said about expanding your idea of sex. I get what you're saying and when Audre Lorde is like, "the uses of the erotic ..." but sometimes I'm like, "Audre, you like to cum too, right?" Like, it wasn't just like, "I feel really turned on about liberation and shit." [Laughing] But at the same time, I do think that there's a lot that's important about just expanding our concepts of sexuality, and I think that crips do that so much anyways when our bodies are different.

One thing that we're trying to do with this project of writing Crip Sex Moments[37] is like ... I don't know, I kind of think of it as like: the good, the bad, the ugly, and the real. You know? Because I feel like there's the good stuff, that's like the secrets of like, wow, the ways that we find to have really amazing hot sex in our bodies is incredible and the kind of like cross-crip solidarity through *fucking*. Maybe you're fucking someone who has your exact disability; maybe they have a different one. But even though you don't have the same experience, you're giving each other love and appreciation and you're like, "Wow you're really fucking hot and I'm gonna figure out how to make you feel pleasure in your body and I'm gonna respect your body and you're gonna do the same thing, awesome."

---

37 "Crip Sex Moments" was a series of interwoven performance pieces telling disabled sex stories E.T. Russian and I wrote for Sins Invalid's 2011 show. Mine are included in *Bodymap*, my 2015 collection of poetry.

PART
II

CRIPPING THE APOCALYPSE

SOME OF MY WILD DISABILITY JUSTICE DREAMS

EVERYONE LOVES DISABILITY JUSTICE; NO ONE WANTS TO DO IT

Sick and disabled and neurodivergent folks aren't supposed to dream, especially if we are queer and Black or brown—we're just supposed to be grateful the "normals" let us live. But I am the product of some wild disabled Black and brown queer revolutionary dreaming, and I am dedicated to dreaming more sick and disabled queer brown femme dreams in 2018.

It's been thirteen years since the original Disability Justice Collective—made up of activists Patty Berne, Leroy Moore, Mia Mingus, Sebastian Margaret, and Eli Clare, a group of disabled people holding a variety of Black, Asian, white, queer, and trans identities—came together to coin the term "disability justice" and lay the groundwork for a movement-building framework of intersectional, revolutionary disability politics.

And right now, we're at an interesting moment in the history of disability justice. It's one where white disabled people who are the reason we invented disability justice because they've ignored or actively excluded disabled Black and brown people for decades are saying, "Hey, that's a fun term" and slapping "disability justice" on their all-white crip conference or panel. It's also a moment in which, as Sins Invalid cofounder Patty Berne said in 2015, "In recent years, on websites and new media locales, on flyers and in informal conversations, I've witnessed people add the word 'justice' onto virtually everything disability related—from disability rights based services and access audits to disability scholarship—while doing nothing to shift either process or end goal, thinking that the word change alone brings that work into alignment with disability justice."[38]

I agree. I've noticed tons of abled activists will happily add "ableism" to the list of stuff they're against (you know, like that big sign in front of the club in my town that says "No racism, sexism, homophobia, transphobia, ableism") or throw around the word "disability justice" in the list of "justices" in their manifesto. But then nothing else changes: all their organizing is still run the exact same inaccessible way, with the ten-mile-long marches, workshops that urge people to "get out of your seats and move!" and lack of inclusion of any disabled issues or organizing strategies. And of course none of them think they're ableist. Kicking cripples down the street? They'd never do that! They're just totally clueless about what disability justice is or, indeed, what disability is, and that it's not bad. They still silently believe that they'd rather die than be us, think of disabled, sick, or crazy people as "flaky" or "inspirational" but also pathetic and gross, don't know any disabled history, and are still running shit the exact same way that makes or forces most of us to stay home.

Many abled Black and brown activists I know remain ignorant of the fact that sick and disabled Black and brown people are doing critical organizing and cultural work on issues from protesting the police murders of Black and brown disabled people to not being killed off by eugenics, killer cops, and medical neglect, from fighting the end of the Affordable Care Act, Medicaid, and the Americans with Disabilities Act to claiming the right to exist as we are.

No matter how much shit I post on Instagram about it, they seem to remain ignorant of the fact that we have histories and cultures and

---

38   Patty Berne, "Disability Justice: A Working Draft," *Sins Invalid*, June 10, 2015, http://sinsinvalid.org/blog/disability-justice-a-working-draft-by-patty-berne, accessed June 18, 2018.

skills and visions, and that if we're going to survive the Trumpocalypse and make the new world emerge, our work needs to be *cripped the fuck out*. Our work needs to center disability justice and the activists at the core of it, where being sick, disabled, mad, neurodivergent/autistic and/or Deaf is at the heart of our radicalism.

THE CRIP ART OF FAILURE: BASED ON REAL-LIFE EVENTS

Recently, on a conference call, a totally well-meaning able-bodied person asked me: "We just have one question! Uh ... What is disability justice? Like, how do we do it?"

I said something diplomatic, like you do when you're trying to keep a gig you need. But in my head, I laughed my ass off. In my head I was like, *You wanna know how you'll know if you're doing disability justice? You'll know you're doing it because people will show up late, someone will vomit, someone will have a panic attack, and nothing will happen on time because the ramp is broken on the supposedly "accessible" building. You won't meet your benchmarks on time, or ever. We won't be grateful to be included; we will want to set the agenda. And what our leadership looks may include long sick or crazy leaves, being nuts in public, or needing to empty an ostomy bag and being on Vicodin at work. It is slow. It's people even the most social justice-minded abled folks stare at or get freaked out by. It looks like what many mainstream abled people have been taught to think of as failure.*

Disability justice, when it's really happening, is too messy and wild to really fit into traditional movement and nonprofit industrial complex structures, because our bodies and minds are too wild to fit into those structures. Which is no surprise, because nonprofits, while created in the '60s to manage dissent, in many ways overlap with "charities"—the network of well-meaning institutions designed on purpose to lock up, institutionalize, and "help the handicapped." Foundations have rarely ever given disabled people money to run our own shit. Nonprofits need us as clients and get nervous about us running the show. Disability justice means the show has to change—or get out of the way.

It's so easy to look at a list of disability justice principles and nod your head. But the real deal is messy and beautiful and real, as messy and beautiful and real as our bodyminds. And it's always something I can't quite get across when abled folks ask me what the hell I'm talking about. It's more like:

> You and your friend are stressed out about Trump so you plan a show about how our disabled Black and brown ancestors survived fascism. They have a traumatic brain injury, and dealing with forms and email is hard for them, so you write a successful grant to the city arts commission in six hours with your ND hyperfocus brain. You get overwhelmed and aphasic by multiple people talking at the same time, but they don't, so they're the one who takes the lead on doing tech and preshow production tasks. The gay theater's staff are nice but pretty overworked, and you end up doing a lot more of the production work than you bargained for. Artists are interested, but it's like herding cats to get some of them to respond to your emails inviting them to be in the show. When you talk with them, it turns out that a lot of them feel huge impostor syndrome about being disabled intersectional artists, are terrified they aren't "real artists" and need a lot of support. Your co-coordinator has a really hard time getting the ASL interpreters to write back and then books them for all four nights. When you get the bill, the ASL rate is three times as high as you budgeted because the agency refused to give a quote. The livestream dies halfway through, and someone gets pissed on Facebook because

*they're homebound and can't see the show now. You blow
out an ovarian cyst on day two and are in a lot of pain
but still have to emcee the show, but you ask for help and
people come through. Despite this, at the end of it all, you
and your friend still love each other and everyone says the
show was amazing. And also, when you are $1,200 short
on the ASL, a) a former DJ collective that went bust due to
internal drama gives you some money that's leftover in their
bank account and b) a community member wins a huge
settlement against SSDI and gives you $250 in cash from
the ATM outside their building, because you helped them
stay housed last year by passing the hat at the last show.*

Disability is a set of innovative, virtuosic skills. When abled
people fuss about how hard it is to make access happen, I laugh and
think about the times I've stage-managed a show while having a panic
attack, or the time the accessible van with three wheelchair-using
performers and staff inside broke and we just brainstormed for two
hours—*Maybe if we pull another van up and lower their ramp onto the
busted ramp folks can get out? Who has plywood? If we go to the bike
shop, will they have welding tools?*—until we figured out a way to fix
the ramp so they could get out. If we can do this, why can't anybody?

And this innovation, this persistence, this commitment to not
leaving each other behind, the power of a march where you move as
slowly as the slowest member and put us in the front, the power of a
lockdown of scooter users in front of police headquarters, the power
of movements that know how to bring each other food and medicine
and organize from tired without apology and with a sense that tired
people catch things people moving fast miss—all of these are skills
we have. I want us to know that—abled and disabled.

DISABILITY JUSTICE IS ABOUT BUILDING RELATIONSHIPS

Over the past decade, I've seen many a well-meaning abled person or organization read a bunch of shit on the internet, follow the access guides, and do all the right things—get the accessible space, book an ASL interpreter, and ask people to be fragrance-free—and then be surprised and also kind of miffed when disabled, Deaf, sick, and mad folks don't show up en masse.

It shouldn't be so hard to figure out why this is: the abled people in question don't know any actual disabled, Deaf, neurodivergent, or Mad folks, or think that they don't, that "they" (us) are somewhere out there. Ableism and audism structurally separate disabled and Deaf people from abled and hearing folks. Literally. It's hard to make friends when the bar you always go to has a flight of stairs, you're meeting until two a.m., and/or you don't know the language of the person you're trying to talk to.

When abled people get ASL and ramps and fragrance-free lotion but haven't built relationships with any disabled people, it just comes off like the charity model once again—*Look at what we're doing for you people! Aren't you grateful?* No one likes to be included as a favor. Inclusion without power or leadership is tokenism.

When I see disability justice flourishing, it comes from years of relationship building and building trust, from fucking up, making repair, learning from mistakes, and showing up for each other. In Toronto, hearing disabled people and Deaf people built relationships with each other for years, including creating community-controlled queer ASL classes so hearing crips could communicate with D(d)eaf and Hard of Hearing queers, resulting in powerful community connections. That didn't happen by accident. It happened because disabled and Deaf people organized together, showed up at each other's protests. When hearing disabled people learn ASL so they can communicate with Deaf folks, we are creating the rock-bottom tools we need to talk, laugh, hang out, disagree, organize, break isolation, and fall in love. And that is the opposite of a well-meaning but relationshipless access provision.

ABLED PEOPLE: TIME'S UP. ESPECIALLY BECAUSE YOU WILL EVENTUALLY BECOME US

It would be easy for me to write the same article that many sick, disabled, Deaf, and mad/ neurodivergent folks before me have written to the abled—asking the abled to get it the fuck together and stop "forgetting" about access and disabled demands. It would be easy for me to write because it's still so needed: non-disabled activists of color continue to "forget" about basic access at events and meetings until someone disabled bugs them about it—or they remember for a few months after a workshop, or a year, and then the issue fades in importance again.

It breaks my heart every time, but besides not wanting to grieve being forgotten, at the end of the day, I'm practical: I want to win! If movements got it together about ableism, there is so much we could win—movement spaces where elders, parents, and sick and disabled folks (a huge amount of the planet) could be present—strength in numbers! We could create movement spaces where people don't "age out" of being able to be involved after turning forty or feel ashamed of admitting any disability, Crazyness, or chronic illness. We could create visions of revolutionary futures that don't replicate eugenics—where disabled people exist and are thriving, not, as often happens in abled revolutionary imaginations, revolutionary futures where winning the rev means we don't exist anymore because everyone has health care.

So, I will say, once: I want abled people to get it together in 2018. Stop forgetting about disability and access. Read some of the many brilliant, made-by-disabled-people access guides out there. Normalize access and disability. Learn about disabled cultures and histories. Look at the histories of disability in your own family and communities. Ask how you are fighting ableism in every campaign you do. Don't forget about us. Realize you are or will be us.

WILD DISABILITY JUSTICE DREAMS AND UNPACKING SHAME

My wild dreaming has me longing to go deeper than just getting basic access. As my friend and comrade Stacey Milbern recently posted on Facebook, "Sometimes I feel impatient about how much ableism has forced us to emphasize accessibility ... [But access] is only the first step in movement building. People talk about access as the outcome, not the process, as if having spaces be accessible is enough to get us all free. Disabled people are so much more than our access needs; we can't have a movement without safety and access, and yet there is so much more still waiting for us collectively once we build this skillset of negotiating access needs with each other."

Going deeper than basic access in our disability justice revolution as Black, Indigenous, and brown people isn't simple. It means unpacking our deep histories of scarcity and shame. Sometimes when disabled people of color bring up access needs, I see able-bodied comrades of color's faces turn stony and shut down. This often does not just come from a casual hatred of sick and disabled people, though that exists too. But sometimes, a person who's angry and defensive about an inaccessible space is flashing back to their mom who died poor and alone, their uncle's polio or schizophrenia no one would talk about, the way the only survival story many Black and brown communities have had is to deny our needs, work sixteen hours, and suck it up. Many of us hold stories about how our families survived enslavement, colonization, and other forms of violence's grueling physical labor by not being disabled. Disabled people in those stories didn't make it—they got killed. Many of us were taught from a young age that care, softness, and healing were for other people, and we needed to just make it work. We sit in legacies of scarcity, survival, and deep, unpacked grief that sometimes make people bitter and enraged when they see someone asking, as if they have a goddamn right to, for a chair, a moment, a bathroom that works.

I've also worked with many organizations—hell, I've been a part of them—where having no money was both the norm and something we prided ourselves on knowing how to make work and look beautiful. We could make a twenty-four-city action happen on a quarter tank of gas and no sleep. We didn't have money to pay ourselves for the hundreds of hours of work we did; every space said no to us, so we made do with the one queer bar or APIA community center space we had. And when someone showed up pointing out that the space was up a flight of stairs, or asked if there was ASL, or wanted some kind of fragrance-free product, we often met them with a mix of bitterness and rage. *We're not even paying ourselves and you want what??? My grandmother worked in the fields all her life; she never had an "access need."*

There is grief mixed in with the rage, and survival, and a belief that you must be spoiled or entitled to ask for what you need. It reminds me of survivors who stubbornly insist that their parents beat them and they came out just fine. I honor the survival skills of denying need and getting the fuck by have been things that kept us alive. But I believe our beloved dead want us to do more than life on one cracker and an inaccessible building, forever. I also believe that we have other lineages of sick and disabled Black and brown ancestors, and non-disabled ones other than "The cripples got left to die; only the strong survived." Before colonization, enslavement, and disaster, we had cultures where disability was a normal part of human existence, where we were honored and valued. As Black disabled queer writer and organizer Cyree Jarelle Johnson remarked to me, "Harriet Tubman had seizures and narcolepsy because a slave owner threw a weight at her head. While on trips she likely had to sit down, lay down, move slowly and rest. Her comrades didn't abandon her then, and we can figure out how not to abandon each other now."39

We have ancestral shame to heal. We have disabled lineages to honor. Let's get to it.

LET'S LIVE LONG, BEAUTIFUL, CRIPPED-OUT LIVES

I know more than one genius organizer—usually a Black or brown sick or disabled woman or nonbinary person who doesn't have a ton of disability community—who's casually told me that they'll be dead by the age of fifty. I respect that crip years are like dog years, and sometimes we live really huge lives in short amounts of time, but I can't help but think that it doesn't have to be that way. We're soaked since birth in narratives that we will die young, that our lives aren't worth living, and that we're up against everything from insurance denials to police trying to kill us who want to do the same damn thing.

But as I hear my friends talking about how they're sure they'll die young, I wonder if changing the narratives around care might change their expectations of dying young. I think about what it would take to continue to build communities of care, where caring for each other is something we actually practice and build the structures to hold. I think of Loree Erickson's mutual aid care collective and how it is both a model of being cared for when the state fails and a place so many people in Toronto get brought into disabled community that is deeply joyful, sexy, and fun in a way that many people don't think of when they think of care. When I try to explain the care collective to folks outside Toronto, there's a silence—it's because they can't quite imagine someone asking for and receiving help, including help that sees you naked and helps you with intimate acts, without shame and with joy. And I wonder—how would our belief that we could live rich,

---

39 Cyree Jarelle Johnson, personal communication with the author, May 15, 2018.

long disabled lives worth living change if we created more mutual aid collectives?

And I also think of the complexities of receiving care. I love collective care—but I would be lying if I said that it was simple, or the sole answer. I think about the many people I know and love who have a really hard time receiving care because "care" has always been conditional, or violent—the invasion of social workers or Child Protective Services or psychiatrists with the power to lock you up. I think about the need for care that can be accessed when you're isolated, disliked, and without social capital—which many disabled people are. I think about how power dynamics and abuse can creep into the most well-meaning care collectives of friends, and of my friends who need twelve to fifteen hours of care a day, which is difficult to impossible for most unpaid friends to provide. I think about the person I was lovers with who was an asshole about thirty percent of that time, who I still send twenty bucks every now and then because they are seriously disabled and can't work. I do this because they are a queer and trans person of color who grew up working class who's pissed off a lot of people, and they still don't deserve to die alone in their own piss. I think about my friend who said, "I never want my ability to go to the bathroom to be dependent on how liked I am." I think about how relieved I was to discover that the state I live in offered twenty-four hours of emergency respite care to caregivers—someone well paid by the state who could come in and pick up meds, do some home care, and fold laundry—that my partner and I could access if one or both of us had a medical crisis. I think of the disability networks where friends and total strangers on the internet bring each other soup and share meds and send money and how lifesaving that is—and what happens when someone is kicked out of that Facebook group.

Recently, Stacey Milbern brought up the concept of "crip doulas"—other disabled people who help bring you into disability community or into a different kind of disability than you may have experienced before. The more seasoned disabled person who comes and sits with your new crip self and lets you know the hacks you might need, holds space for your feelings, and shares the community's stories. She mentioned that it's telling that there's not even a word for this in mainstream English. We wondered together: How would it change people's experiences of disability and their fear of becoming disabled if this were a word, and a way of being? What if this was a rite of passage, a form of emotional labor folks knew of—this space of helping people transition? I have done this with hundreds of people. What if this is something we could all do for each other? How would our movements change? Our lives? Our beliefs about what we can do?

CRIPPING THE APOCALYPSE
WE'VE ALREADY SURVIVED THE END OF THE WORLD

2017 felt apocalyptic. One place I felt the apocalypse was in the wildfires that covered the Pacific Northwest. One morning, I went outside and the air was dark gray. Something gray was sprinkling from the sky. Was it ... ash?

At first, the people on the news were optimistic. It should be over in a day. Then a week. Then maybe next week we'd have breathable air.

The news reports trickled in: fueled by climate change, giant wildfires in British Columbia had spread to cover most of Washington State. Fires started in the Columbia River basin near Portland. Then fires came to Santa Rosa and Southern California. Everyone was coughing and stressed out. I canceled a planned writing retreat in Northern California because I was scared of driving through fires circling the highway.

And when the texts started to come in—*Hey, is anyone else feeling like they can't breathe, like they're sick from all the smoke? Am I making a big deal out of nothing, or is the smoke making me feel super foggy?*—who were the people who already knew about masks, detox herbs, air purifiers, and somatic tricks for anxiety?

Yeah, you guessed it. Over and over, it was sick and disabled folks—particularly folks with chemical injuries, environmental illness, asthma, and other autoimmune conditions who had been navigating unsafe air for years—sharing the knowledge that being sick and disabled had already taught us. We had comprehensive information about where to get masks and respirators and about the right herbs to take to detox after exposure to air pollutants. We knew to go to libraries and other air-conditioned places to get an air break. We knew about HEPA filters and how you can make one with a furnace filter and a box fan. We knew it was normal to feel fatigue, confusion, and panic, and we knew to hit inhalers and take antianxiety herbs. Lightning Bolt,[40] a disability justice activist group formed in the wake of Trump to do community-based trainings around access and community safety without the police, led a successful Masks to the People campaign, crowdfunding money to buy masks that they distributed to people living in tent cities in the Bay Area, since people living outside walls are extremely vulnerable to toxic smoke.

Since Trump got elected, many people in my community have been talking about how Octavia Butler was a prophet and how her books *Parable of the Sower* and *Parable of the Talents* eerily predicted the climate change, wildfires, and fascism of our current world. Many people in movement spaces have taken Butler's words as prophecy and text. (I'm not hating on that conversation: full disclosure, as one of the writers in *Octavia's Brood,* a wildly popular anthology of visionary social justice science fiction in the lineage of Octavia Butler, I've been a part of it.)

But what is often missing from these discussions is how Lauren Olamina, Butler's Black, genderqueer teenage hero who leads her

---

40 https://www.lightningbolt.vision

community out of the ashes and founds a new spirituality that embraces change as god, is disabled.[41] In the book, she is called a sharer: someone with hyperempathy syndrome from her mother's use of the Einstein drug, a popular drug that heightened intelligence. She feels everything everyone feels, and it's often overwhelming in a way that reminds me of some autistic and neurodivergent realities. It gives her impairments and also gifts.

To me, Butler's *Parable* books are a Black disability justice narrative. Lauren often struggles with her nonnormative mind, but it also gives her Black disabled brilliance. Her hyperempathy makes her refuse to leave anyone behind, even when they are a pain in the ass or she disagrees with them. It allows her to innovate, making her survival pack filled with seeds, maps, and money when everyone else thinks she is crazy, cocreating a resistance community and rebuilding it when it's destroyed.

For years awaiting this apocalypse, I have worried that as sick and disabled people, we will be the ones abandoned when our cities flood. But I am dreaming the biggest disabled dream of my life—dreaming not just of a revolutionary movement in which we are not abandoned but of a movement in which we lead the way. With all of our crazy, adaptive-deviced, loving kinship and commitment to each other, we will leave no one behind as we roll, limp, stim, sign, and move in a million ways towards cocreating the decolonial living future.

I am dreaming like my life depends on it. Because it does.

---

41   When I wrote this essay, I had not yet read the brilliant work of Dr Sami Schalk, whose book *Bodyminds Reimagined: (Dis)ability, Race, and Gender in Black Women's Speculative Fiction* goes into much more detail about reading Octavia Butler's *Parable* books through a Black disability framework. Please go read it.

A MODEST PROPOSAL FOR A FAIR TRADE EMOTIONAL LABOR ECONOMY

(CENTERED BY DISABLED, FEMME OF COLOR, WORKING-CLASS/POOR GENIUS)

Femme: A person who has one of a million kinds of queer femme or feminine genders. Part of a multiverse of femme-gendered people, who have histories and communities in every culture since the dawn of time. Often complicated remixes that break away from white, able-bodied, upper-middle-class, cis femininity, remixing it to harken to fat or working class or Black or brown or trans or nonbinary or disabled or sex worker or other genders of femme to grant strength, vulnerability, and power to the person embodying them.

The thing about being a working-class or poor and/or disabled and/or parenting and/or Black, Indigenous, or brown femme is that people are going to ask you to do stuff for them. Oh, are they ever.

They're going to ask you to listen, do a favor, do an errand, drop everything to go buy them some cat food or crisis-counsel them. Manage logistics, answer feelings emails, show up, empathize, build and maintain relationships. Organize the childcare, the access support, the food. Be screamed at, de-escalate, conflict resolute. They're going to say, "Can I just pick your brain about something?" and then send you a five-paragraph email full of pretty goddamn complex questions. It'd be real nice if you could get back to them ASAP. They're going to ask if you can email them your powerpoint and all your resources.

Some of them will be people who are close to you; some of them will be total strangers. *Do you have a minute?*

For free.

Forever.

And you know what's going to happen? You're going to do those things. Because you do, indeed, care. Because it's the right thing to do. Because you're good at it. Because you want to.

And because: your life as a working-class or poor and/or sex-working and/or disabled and/or Black or brown femme person has taught you that the only damn way you or anybody survives is by helping each other. No institutions exist to help us survive—we survive because of each other. Your life is maintained by a complex, nonmonetary economy of shared, reciprocal care. You drop off some extra food; I listen to you when you're freaking out. You share your car with me; I pick you up from the airport. We pass the same twenty dollars back and forth between each other, building movements and communities as we go. It's maybe what hippies mean when they talk about the gift economy; it's just a million times more working-class, femme, Black and brown, and sick in bed.

We live in a white, capitalist, colonialist, ableist patriarchy that oppresses in many ways. One of them is that femininity is universally reviled. Patriarchy, racism, transmisogyny, colonialism, ableism, classism, and whorephobia come together to dish out hate to folks who are femme or feminine in extra fun ways. In the queer communities I have been a part of since the 1990s, I have witnessed over and over how femmephobia, sexism, and transmisogyny act together to view femininity and femmeness as weak, less than, not as smart or competent, "hysterical," "too much," and not as worthy of praise or respect. Forget femme invisibility; the thing most femmes I know are impacted by is lack of femme respect. Femmephobia and transmisogyny infuse queer and mainstream cultures in a million ways, from the ways in which femme genders are seen as inherently less radical and more capitalist/assimilationist (assuming money spent on makeup and dresses is somehow more capitalist than money spent on bow ties and butch hair wax) to the ways in which, as writer Morgan M. Page notes, "any minor slip of language or politics and [trans women] are labeled 'crazy trans women' by cis people while trans men nod knowingly in agreement," resulting in trans women being shunned and expelled from community.

Generations of femmes of many genders have written and organized about misogyny and transmisogyny in queer and trans communities, and I'm able to suck in a deep breath of air now and then because of this work.

But I remain, with many other femme and feminine people, harmed by misogyny—where endless free care work and emotional labor is simply the role my community and the world has for us. We are supposed to wipe the asses of the world without ceasing. As a newly physically disabled, working-class femme of color in the 1990s, I often felt how the queer and radical prison justice communities I was part of looked down upon my gender, especially when I was disabled and broke and surviving abuse and needing support. Then I really sucked—I was just another needy, weak *girl*, huh? The one place femme people could receive respect in those communities was if we were tough, invulnerable, always "on," and never needing a thing. I know I'm not alone, and I know this experience has not ended.

The working-class and poor femmes, Black and brown femmes, sick and disabled femmes, parenting femmes and sex-working and rural femmes I know hold it the fuck down. We pull off shit—from organizing complex marches and transformative justice actions to the life-support work of making sure people are fed, don't die, and don't get evicted—on no sleep and low spoons and a quarter tank of gas, over and over again.

Our organizing skills in these departments are incredible, and often not valued as much as masculine or charismatic leadership, or indeed seen as skills. I want our skills and competency to be respected and rewarded. What I think is a problem is when this labor both becomes the *only* way femmes are rewarded in community and isn't seen as a choice but as what you're just supposed to do (because you're femme, right?). This expectation can be voiced as a veiled or direct compliment—*You're so competent, right? You're so good at this, of course we wanted to ask you*—but it doesn't make the work itself less, well, a gendered demand to work a whole lot. When you're in this gendered situation, you're also presumed to be endlessly available and interruptible. People ask you for help or labor, and "no" is nowhere in their conception of what your response might be. Far too often, the emotional labor we do as femmes or feminine people is not seen as labor—it's seen as air. It's that little thing you do on the side. Not real organizing, not real work, just talking about feelings and buying groceries. Girl stuff. Femme stuff. Disabled and sick stuff, not a real activist holding a big meeting stuff. Thanks, though! That was really helpful!

Before I go any further, I want to be really clear about a few things: I don't think that only femme or feminine people offer care labor, or can. I know femmes who suck at this stuff. And I know many masculine and other-gendered people who do care labor, and I want all genders of people to be receiving and providing that labor in our communities. I've heard masculine folks talk about ways the gendered nature of care labor affects them—from being expected to always be physically super-able-bodied and strong to being expected to be "the rock" that will always be there, without having needs of their own. From Black and brown and working-class and poor men and masculine people being seen through a racist, classist lens that is surprised when they are loving and caring, parenting, and doing care work to disabled masculine people being impacted by complex ways that disability is feminized and denied disabled bodily autonomy. What I want to tease out and focus on are the ways that misogyny, femmephobia, and transmisogyny come together to royally screw over femme people of many genders; how misogyny, femmephobia, and transmisogyny are part of global systems of gender that extract a hell of a lot of labor and energy from femme and feminized people, from parenting and caretaking being considered "free labor" to sexist assumptions of femme perma-availability being made in queer and trans communities. Also, the gendered wage gap is real. Cis and trans women really do get paid less than cis men, and women and femmes who are racialized, disabled, imprisoned and institutionalized, trans, rural and poor/working class get paid extra bad.

Second, I'm not against care work existing. I love the care and mutual aid we give each other in queer, trans, sick and disabled and working class and queer and trans Black, Indigenous, and people of color (QTBIPOC) communities. As a sick and disabled, working-class, brown femme, I wouldn't be alive without communities of care, and neither would most people I love. Some of my fiercest love is reserved for how femmes and sick and disabled queers show up for each other when every able-bodied person "forgets" about us. Sick and disabled folks will get up from where we've been projectile vomiting for the past eight hours to drive a spare Effexor to their friend's house who just ran out. We do this because we love each other, and because we often have a sacred trust not to forget about each other. Able-bodied people who think we are "weak" have no idea; every day of our disabled lives is like an Ironman triathlon. Disabled, sick, poor, working-class, sex-working and Black and brown femmes are some of the toughest and most resilient folks I know. You have to develop complex strengths to survive this world as us.

I love how working-class, femme, and disabled this care labor is. I just want it to also not be seen as an automatic expectation of any femme at any time! I want some rules so we don't feel drained, exhausted, and fucked over. I want it to be a choice. And I want its next-level genius of skill to be recognized. This is skilled labor!

So I would like to advance the radical notion that providing care is work. By work, I mean it's just that: *work*. I mean that the care work we give is essential to building movements that are accessible and sustainable. We are building and maintaining movements when we're texting to make sure someone is okay, talk on the phone for hours, talk shit on the couch, drop off a little care. Those things are not a sideline or an afterthought to our movements. They *are* our movements. And I have seen some of the most femme movements and communities—disabled ones, sex-working ones—organize very differently because they are fully centered around feminized, sick survivor care labor.

I tried an experiment recently. For one week, I logged how many times I was asked for care labor or support, and what I noticed about who was doing the asking, and how. My findings? Every single—really— femme person who hit me up started their requests by asking me how I was doing and prefaced their requests by saying things like, "Hey, if you have time," "Do you have the capacity to give some support?" or "When and if you have time ..." They also were more likely to offer to buy me lunch, trade me for something, run an errand, or pay me. And they were more graceful and heard it the first time when I said, "Hey, I'm so sorry, but I can't right now."

Masculine and non-femme friends, however, were much more likely to just hit me up and say, "Hey, could you ...": pray for them, hook them up with a publisher, tell them what doctor they should go to, listen to them vent about an intense transformative justice process gone wrong, be a reference, or answer a question. It was not uncommon for these requests to come from someone I had not heard from for months. There was no, "Do you think you have the time or spoons to do this?" no suggestion of "I could offer X thing in return," and no "If you don't, it's totally okay." There was also no, "How are you doing?"

This pissed me off. I also knew I was far from alone. My conversations with other femme people are full of us describing our care labor—and of us bitching about how exploited, unappreciated, and exhausted we often feel when that labor isn't recognized. The sexism and femme oppression in these dynamics loom huge. Disabled, white, working-class femme poet Tara Hardy recently remarked at *ADEPT*, a sick and disabled queer performance at Gay City, Seattle's queer theater, "Femmes get objectified two ways, one sexually, the other as Mommy." In the sexist world, Mommy does a million hours of unpaid labor a week without anyone asking them.

There's been a huge amount of writing about emotional labor in the past few years—everything from the oft-reposted Metafilter thread on gendered emotional labor that is now fifty single-spaced pages long to essays by queer and trans writers of color like Kai Cheng Thom and Caleb Luna to Ada Hoffman's wonderful essay about autistic practices of emotional labor to a million conversations I've seen and taken part in with friends and comrades. In thinking about the roots and histories of unpaid and unrecognized labor by feminine people, I don't know how to capture their enormity. But I think about movements like Black Women for Wages for Housework and others who fought for the audacious demand that people should get paid wages for the labor of homemaking and parenting the WSCCAP conceives of as "naturally" being unpaid. I think about movements like the National Domestic Workers Alliance's Caring Across Generations campaign, where elders, disabled people, and the personal care workers who support them—many of whom are immigrant, Black, or brown people performing the feminized labor of personal care support work—are organizing together for fair wages and work conditions and for state health and social services departments to raise pay rates allowed for care support workers. I think about how little people working in "pink-collar" fields that are highly feminized like cleaning, caretaking, childcare, waitressing, and service work get paid. I think about my mom, a former waitress, explaining to me when I was seven years old how waitresses are legally paid far under the minimum wage and are dependent on tips to make any kind of money (tips that depend on the femme emotional labor of being seen as sexy, nice, and cute), and how you should either be ready to pay twenty-five percent *minimum* as a tip or you shouldn't go out to eat. (The current minimum waitress wage in Massachusetts is $2.66 an hour. She made a hell of a lot less in the 1960s.) And I think about Black, Indigenous, brown, working-class women's and femme bodies being forced to work for free or for pennies—as enslaved people on plantations, in Export Processing Zone factories in Sri Lanka and many other Global South countries, and beyond. I think about disabled and Mad people locked in nursing homes and institutions working for well under minimum wage in "sheltered workshops," and I think about people in prison working for pennies an hour. Finally, I think about the rage and oppression many sex workers face for having the gall to actually charge for sexual, emotional labor! It's impossible to think and talk about emotional labor, care work, and gender without talking and thinking about all these intertwined histories and realities of oppression and resistance.

All of this has started me thinking about what the solutions might be. If care labor is, well, labor, and we participate in an emotional economy all the time, what would a just care labor economy look and feel like? What would I want to get paid (in money or care labor or appreciation), and how? What would I want the conditions of my labor to be, to feel that my work was in safe, compensated conditions that had my worker's rights at the center?

This is what I've got. This is just the beginning, but every revolution has to start somewhere. These thoughts are an experiment and a work in progress. Feel free to add your own.

Fair trade emotional economics are consensual. In a fair trade femme care emotional labor economy, there would no unconsensual expectations of automatic caretaking/mommying. People would ask first and be prepared to receive a yes, no, or maybe. I ask if you can offer care or support; you think about whether you've got spoons and offer an honest yes, no, or maybe. In this paradigm, it's the person offering care's job to figure out and keep figuring out what kind of care and support they can offer. It's the person receiving care's job to figure out what they need and what they can accept, under what circumstances. Both folks might need some support and rumination to figure this out. You can negotiate: You can say, "I can't do that, but I could offer this." I can say, "I appreciate that offer, but I think I need someone who can just listen right now." And, most of all, no is okay. I can say, "Honey, I wish I could, but I'm tapped out right now—is there someone else you can talk to?"

Fair trade care webs draw on sick and disabled knowledge about care. Sick and disabled folks have many superpowers: one of them is that many of us have sophisticated, highly developed skills around negotiating and organizing care. Many sick and disabled people have experienced receiving shitty, condescending, "poor you!" charity-based care that's worse than no care at all—whether it's from medical staff or our friends and families. Many disabled people also face receiving abusive or coercive care, in medical facilities and nursing homes and from our families and personal care assistants. We're also offered unsolicited medical advice, from doctors and strangers on the street (who are totally sure carrot juice will cure our MS) every day of our lives. All of those offers are "well meaning," but they're also intrusive, unasked for, and mostly coming from a place of discomfort with disability and wanting to "fix" us.

The idea of consent in care labor is radical and comes from our experiences receiving these kinds of clusterfucks of so-called care. On sick and disabled internet gathering places I hang out in, it's a common practice for folks to ask before they offer advice, or to specify when they're not asking for solutions or tips—or, when they are, what specific kinds of information they're open to. For many, it's mind-blowing that disabled and sick people get to decide for ourselves the kind of care we want and need, and say no to the rest. Ableism mandates that disabled and sick people are always "patients," broken people waiting to be fixed by medicine or God, and that we're supposed to be grateful for anything anyone offers at any time. It is a radical disability justice stance that turns the ableist world on its ear, to instead work from a place where disabled folks are the experts on our own bodies and lives, and we get to consent, or not. We're the bosses of our own bodyminds. This has juicy implications for everyone, including abled people.

Fair trade femme disabled care webs are reciprocal. Recently, my friend Chanelle Gallant commented on Femme Secret Society, a Facebook femme community-building and support group, "Sometimes when I get hit up for advice & support from folks I'm not already friends with, I prefer if they offer me something in exchange. If we are in the same city & what they're asking for will take me hours [to do], I might ask them if they can make me a meal." She asked femmes in the group what kinds of things—including cash—they had asked for as compensation for requests of our free labor. And femmes talked about asking for food, services, pet care, tarot readings, personal services, or bodywork in exchange for emails from strangers that began, "Can I just pick your brain for a minute?" or big, complicated requests for emotional support.

Hearing Gallant and other femmes talk about asking for something in exchange for our emotional labor was a game changer. I had rarely considered asking for something in return for the endless stream of requests for information, mentoring, and support that came into my inbox. Informally, especially in disabled and femme communities I was part of, there was certainly often an unwritten rule that if you gave care, you got some back—it was just good manners. In many Black and brown communities, this all seemed to go along with the concept of good manners or just how you were raised to treat people, what some folks I know call home training. I picked my friend up from the airport and he slept on my couch when he was on tour, and when I was on tour in his city, he offered me the same thing back. But sometimes I just gave a lot and was left exhausted without getting anything back. Not even a thank-you.

Many, many things shifted in my life when I started to think of my care labor as labor, not just "the right thing to do" or "I'll just answer their question, it'll only take a minute." When I started thinking about how much free work I could afford to offer, and if there might be some things I'd like in return.

Everything doesn't have to be fifty-fifty all the time. I think that's especially important for folks who need a lot of care to survive, who may not be able to offer a ton back all the time. But I would argue for a general bend towards offering something back, even just a thank-you, a "Hey, I see the work you just put in" or a "I'm too sick to do anything right now, but I can offer this when I can." Shit, I had someone give me a ten-dollar jar of fancy kraut they'd shoplifted the other week to thank me for something! It's not good manners to always take and never give back.

Reciprocity of care labor is also a disabled practice. In disabled communities, we talk about the idea that we can still offer reciprocity to each other, even if we can't offer the exact same type of care back. For example: if my disabled body can't lift yours onto the toilet, it doesn't mean I can't be reciprocal—it means I contribute equally from what my particular body can do. Maybe instead of doing physical care, I can research a medical provider, buy groceries for you when I'm out shopping, or listen to you vent when one of your dates was ableist.

Fair trade care labor is not a one-sided, femmephobic, sexist shit show. Masculine and other genders of people can notice feelings and offer to listen and do childcare too! I swear to fucking god, these are learnable skills!

Fair trade care economics could be kinda like ... permaculture? The more systems are not a monoculture, the more sustainable they will be. The more there are a lot of different kinds of folks giving and receiving different kinds of care, the more there's room for boundaries, ebbs and flows, people tapping out, and people moving up. Crips and nonnormative people have a lot of different gifts to offer, and normals and ableds often assume not only that we have nothing to offer, but that we can only be (patronizingly and abusively) cared for. But care doesn't have to be one way. It can become an ongoing responsive ecosystem, where what is grown responds to need.

Vacation, time off, sick time, weekends, and time and a half could be part of the deal. Maybe not exactly the way they are when you work at Target but ... some kind of way? A fair trade disabled femme working-class emotional care economy would give people doing emotional labor time off. We would get to have limits to our hyper-responsibility. We would get to have lives that are more than bouncing from crisis response to crisis response.

Because we deserve joy and rest. And while crisis and extreme states are common parts of human experience when we have just gone through a really hard slog—being there for someone who is suicidal or negotiating an intense death in the community—in this economic system, it's not just okay, it's accepted and normal to not run to the next crisis after we've just finished one but, instead to ask someone else to move up and take the baton.

Disabled femme fair trade emotional economics receives a thank-you. Our work is seen as work. Our emotional labor is respected. We are not just asked to labor, and then asked to labor again. We get—dare I say it—appreciation cards and bonuses? I'm not talking about Starbucks gift cards at Christmas, necessarily, and I'm not talking about the kind of forced gratitude that is demanded from many of us in return for care. I am talking about a culture of appreciation, respect, and thank-yous for care that doesn't have to do with groveling or bullshit. I am talking about what many of us already do: notice, thank, and witness the work being done.

Imagine how free we could get if instead of femme labor being an unpaid, demanded mommy tap, we could be thanked and compensated for our work, and then kick back and put our feet up, smiling. Imagine if it was compensated and the labor conditions were fair—maybe everyone would want to do it more. Imagine if we were not only respected for our care labor but also allowed to be more than our care labor.

Imagine how much we could win if there was more than enough care to go around.

PREFIGURATIVE POLITICS AND RADICALLY ACCESSIBLE PERFORMANCE SPACES

MAKING THE WORLD TO COME

> *If, as the African revolutionary leader Amílcar Cabral described it, culture is the "collective personality of a people," then the arts are its collective dreamlife. In the absence of coercive control, the arts, like dreams, are naturally drawn to the deepest hopes, fears, and truths that are suppressed in daily life ... art becomes conscious dream-telling, responsible creation with the potential to affect the life of our people.*
> —Ricardo Levins Morales

Prefigurative politics is a fancy term for the idea of imagining and building the world we want to see now. It's waking up and acting as if the revolution has happened. It's, for example, building a sliding scale community acupuncture clinic that is affordable and centers disabled and working-class/poor and Black, Indigenous, and people of color instead of writing reports about how the medical-industrial complex is fucked up. (Though that can be important too.) I think of it as akin to the Allied Media Conference principles of "We spend more time building than attacking" and "We focus on our power, not our powerlessness."

The higher education programs where I studied writing and performance taught basically zero about creating accessibility in making performance art, theater, and spoken word. The focus was almost always on creating the work of Art, in a vacuum. Almost no attention was paid to the audience, the performance space, the container, and the community for the art as being as important as the art itself, and not separable from the art. Practical skills—from how to make a flyer or a budget to how to do successful ASL and make a fragrance-free space or a performance whose pace was accessible to non–hyper-able-bodied performers—were neglected in those ivory towers. I think that if anyone had asked about how to create accessible spaces, for performers or attendees, they would have been, gently or not so gently, dissed. That stuff, that's about community-based art, or art therapy—not real, professional, capital A art. As a performer and curator/producer, I believe that how you do it and who is there to see it is are as important as what is on the stage. My favorite performance spaces are spaces that become temporary, two-hour communities that are autonomous zones that feel like freedom. Being in them, we can smell and taste and feel things we have always wanted but rarely witnessed—both in what we see on stage and how we interact and participate as an audience that serves as a community of witnesses. Having an accessible space for performers and attendees and workers, where disability is not marginalized, tokenized, or simply absent, is very different from having a performance space that is full of mostly able-bodied, young, non-parenting people who can afford to spend the money to attend and/or to get there in the first place.

As oppressed people, we don't control a lot of things. But one thing we can sometimes control is the stage. The stage can be prefigurative politics.

I often tell a story about Patty Berne, the cofounder and Haitian Japanese femme powerchair-using disabled badass artist and organizer of Sins Invalid. I once asked her why she had chosen to use performance art as her primary way to advance disability justice. Why not just do a workshop? She paused and said, "You know, I could do workshops until I was blue in the face, trying to convince white disabled people or able-bodied people of color to care about us. And I've done that. Or I could make a three-minute piece of performance art that shows them the inside of their dreams and nightmares and fucks their shit up. I chose that route."

Disability, access, and accessibility are rarely thought about in performance. Access is a guilt-ridden afterthought, when it's thought of at all, and it's usually only thought of when disabled people ask about accessibility. This request is usually responded to with guilt, with defensiveness, with surprise, with bad or nonexistent or last-minute scrambles for access, or with simply with abled tears. Because, as Qwo-Li Driskill says, one way ableism works is that disabled people "are not even present within the imaginations of a supposedly radical future."[42]

Further, in ableist, mainstream performance spaces, access is mostly only ever considered—maybe—when audience members are concerned. In my experience, most theater managers and staff never imagine that performers, directors, light and sound techs, stage managers, and volunteers could be disabled. Writing this, I can remember clearly the pause on the other end of the phone when I asked my contact at a performance space whether the stage was accessible, after he'd said, "Oh yeah, there's a ramp at the door" three times, and I'd said, "Yes, but is there a ramp for the *stage?*" He couldn't imagine that one of the performers was a wheelchair user. When he finally got it, he said without hesitation, "Well, I guess she'll just have to perform on the floor," without thinking for a second about the second-class place implied by that state—able-bodied and walkie crips get the stage; you get the floor.

This fucks everybody over, because more access is more access for everyone! Don't get me started about the theater manager who said,

---

42   Qwo-Li Driskill, with Aurora Levins Morales and Leah Lakshmi Piepzna-Samarasinha, "Sweet Dark Places: Letters to Gloria Anzaldúa on Disability, Creativity, and the Coatlicue State," in *El Mundo Zurdo 2: Selected Works from the Society of the Study of Gloria Anzaldúa*, edited by Sonia Saldivar Hull, Norma Alarcon, and Rita E. Urquijo-Ruiz (San Francisco: Aunt Lute, 2012) 75–98.

"Oh yeah, it's accessible" to me on the phone, where we showed up on opening night to find a gorgeous ramp from the green room to the stage, and rejoiced. Two years later, when we showed up again, the ramp was gone. What happened? "Oh, we built it for you because we knew you had someone in a wheelchair, but after your show was over, we tore it down," a staff member explained helpfully—as if this made sense. My friend, Black, wheelchair-using, queer, femme dancer and writer Neve Mazique-Bianco, looked at me levelly when I broke the news and said, "Leah, we just have to remember that the abled will destroy access at all costs." The irony was that nice wide ramp would've helped everyone—people in chairs, people using canes, and normals who just needed to haul a lot of props onstage the way, you know, you usually have to in theater. But there you have it. Oppression isn't helpful or logical.

We are not supposed to be healers, because we are obviously "unhealed" and broken, according to the ablest imagination. And we are not supposed to be performers, except in a "clap for the brave cripples, but don't expect them to be a) good b) have some shocking shit to say that you didn't expect" kind of way. The charity model infects even how crip art can be thought of, or if it can be thought of at all.

Which brings me, though, to the joyous work of setting up performances and what happens when making access happen is not an afterthought to producing performance but a central part of visioning and creating that performance, from the beginning.

Perhaps you've heard the idea that the audience makes the performance. As a performer of color, I know that performing to an all QTBIPOC audience is very different from performing to one that is majority white (or to one where white people have grabbed all the seats right at the front).

The audience at a Sins show is as important as the show. Is part of the show. Because it is a portrait of cross-disabled, deeply accessible space that is also Black, brown, and economically accessible.

When I went to a Sins show for the first time and ran smack into crip culture—a line of chair and scooter users right at the front; a line of Deaf, Hard of Hearing, and signing folks at the front right in front of the 'terps; short folks; cane users; folks with PCAs; folks in pain, dressed up, dressed all in white, popping pills, flirting, spraying active enzymes under their tongues to withstand chemicals they were surrounded by, sitting by audio describers; Black, brown, and white; no one turned away for lack of funds—it fucked me up in the best way and changed my life. This was the audience. I was a part of the audience. A brown, sick part. We were not translating and we were not trying to pass as abled or fighting to just get in the door or to see five seconds of ourselves onstage, and the world was the world to be. And we were not "Sorry, the space is inaccessible, but you can watch it on the livestream!" (Note: I am all in favor of livestreaming as being a way to make performance accessible to folks who are unable to make it to the show because of money, sickness, fatigue, etc., but livestreaming is not an okay fix for an inaccessible venue—sick, disabled, Deaf, and crazy folks would like to be part of the community gathering to witness performance too.) We were not an afterthought. Able-bodied people could come, but they weren't doing us any favors.

Over the next few years, as I grew in disability consciousness and identity, and took part in hanging out, talking, thinking, and building DJ culture with other sick and disabled folks, I started thinking a lot more, and trying to put into practice, accessible booking and producing. I learned a lot from others doing this work.

It took a long time before I realized that the work I was automatically doing as a disabled producer—buying the fragrance-free soap, booking ASL and doing Deaf promo and making sure that everyone got their scripts in to the 'terps two weeks in advance, taping off lanes thirty-six inches wide, figuring out where interpreters, Deaf, and HOH folks could sit near each other and still have clear sight lines, doing preshow education about fragrance-free, recruiting childcare workers, calling venues multiple times to punch through their "Oh yeah, it's accessible" to find out what that really meant, cocreating an accessible venues Google doc—was both a specific skill set of accessible performance skills and its own job that no one should be doing *and* directing, performing, etc. And that it was an invisibilized labor because it is feminized, disabled cultural labor. And it is never taught in a theatrical or performance MFA. And mostly, when it happens, it happens because sick and disabled and Deaf and crazy folks make it happen, because we are the ones who a) care and b) have the sick/disabled/crazy/Deaf science and skills to make it happen.

Five years after I attended that first Sins show, when I was working on booking the Mangos with Chili Toronto show, I listened to myself as I explained that the culture in Toronto had shifted—not at all fully, and not automatically, but through years and decades of cross-disability and Deaf cultural activism in Toronto, and it was no longer just acceptable business as usual all the time to have queer performance in inaccessible spaces. People who did could expect resistance and a community raising our voices in anger. (I say this with hesitation, knowing that there are still so many inaccessible spaces, and that this is an ongoing work in progress—but also wanting to mark that accessibility awareness in Toronto QTBIPOC and activist performance spaces does feel broader than in many cities that I have visited. And that that happened through the labor of many, many disabled, chronically ill, crazy, and Deaf folks and allies, and deserves to be celebrated.)

And I was rewarded. At the show, there was a line of signing folks right up front, parents who were able to watch burlesque because there was childcare on-site, chair users with nice wide rows and clear beginning and end times marked on the invite so Wheel-Trans bookings could happen, frag-free seating, folks who left halfway through because they got too tired, youth, and elders.

That crowd was the show.

And more than that: that crowd was the movement and community I want to live in and make art for and with. It was the opposite of an inaccessible performance space filled with able-bodied, non-parenting, young queers. For three hours, it was a cross-disability, parenting, and mixed-class community where I felt like all my parts could come home. I didn't feel like I was pushing myself to be in a space that was inaccessible, and where the fact of disabled people wasn't even present. I wasn't at home, staying away from an inaccessible and alienating space, worried that I would fade from people's memory or become a "Whatever happened to her?" because I had just stopped going to inaccessible spaces. Where I was not isolated from other disabled, Deaf, chronically ill, and/or Crazy folks because of the walls ableism enacts to separate us from each other and forcibly isolate us.

That show and crowd—it was the world to come.

CHRONICALLY ILL TOURING ARTIST PRO TIPS

Caveat: This works for me. This does not work for all bodies. YMMV (your mileage may vary). Take what works; leave the rest. Write your own too.

I have had fibromyalgia and spinal arthritis for half my life. I am also a touring artist, and that's one of the ways I hack ableism—writing for money and getting college gigs allows me to do some work that makes money in short chunks, and then allows me rest time. However, even if touring is one way of hacking capitalism as a sick weirdo, touring still puts my bodymind through the wringer. Over the past couple decades on cheap planes and buses, I have come up with some hacks that make me feel more cared for and less likely to fall apart. (Or make the falling apart feel less awful.) These might be helpful for you if your immune system is like Swiss cheese, you are tired all the time, smells make you barf and migraine, and the airlines are not nice to you and your mobility devices.

1. Yin chiao. Think your immune system is doing great for once? Think you won't get sick on tour? Think again. You are going to be on college campuses meeting a million students who all give colds to each other, or you're at a community center or bookstore that is the same. You are going to be on a million airplanes and buses, or in a van with twelve people who are having sex with each other, or in a student co-op with questionable dishwashing

practices. You are going to be drinking water and eating food from all kinds of places your body isn't used to, and you will get sick. If you pound yin chiao (three to four pills, three times a day, at the first sign of feeling sick), you might not get *that* sick, or sick at all. Stockpile, as it is not always easy to find outside of health food store land or APIA communities. Astragalus powder or tincture, probiotics (your gut is your first line of immune defense) all help too.

2. Sea salt. Feel that tickle in your throat/Oh shit, I'm getting sick feeling? Hot sea salt gargles, stat. They'll stop the bacteria from going into your lungs. Upper respiratory infections are easier to treat than ones that get in your lungs. You can also throw some in a bath if you have crotch itch. And it'll help ease sore muscles. If you need to do a protection spell, ditto.

3. Melatonin. At some point you will desperately need to sleep, but you will be in Melbourne, Australia, or Grinnell, Iowa, and your body will just be like, "Nope, we like our old time zone!" and you will be fucked, fucked, fucked. You will not be able to sleep, and then you will have to wake up and talk and teach and perform and navigate, and you will have no sleep, and you will cry—but melatonin will knock you out. Benadryl works too, but I like melatonin better.

4. Activated charcoal. Your guts are going to completely fucking rebel against you for deviating from your normal kale taco diet and subsisting off of the Starbucks Perfect Oatmeal cup, yogurt parfaits from the grab-and-go case, jerky, shawarma, and burgers. At some point, you will eat day-old tater tots, and mayo that was in the van a little too long, and you will hurl. These babies will absorb the gas and the badness and stop you from puking on a fifteen-hour Megabus run. Ginger chews or just crystallized

ginger will stop you from puking too, and they are often stocked at bodegas and corner stores.

5. Ibuprofen. Vitamin I. If it doesn't make your stomach bleed, just go ahead and take 800 milligrams (four pills, which are typically 200 milligrams each) every four hours, especially before and after riding in planes and buses. It'll help inflammation go down. Turmeric pills or tea is a great substitute that is easier on the gut.

6. A big scarf. Cold on the plane or bus? Van mates driving you nuts? Can't sleep on the plane? Just need to shut out the world? Put this over your face.

7. Emergency protein. A friend once said, "I'd carry around half a cow if I could." Jerky, almonds, whatever. Wild canned salmon from Trader Joe's is a life-transforming game changer—$3.99 for a big can of cheap, good protein—but it stinks up the van or the plane.

8. Kale salad holds up for at least two days unrefrigerated in a Tupperware if it's not too hot outside. You can also just get a lot of whatever bar you like and keep them at the bottom of your sack.

9. Get a big-ass mason jar, stick half a lemon in it, and fill it up with water once you clear security at the airport. Voilà—electrolytes and hydration. Pick herbs by the curb or from an unsprayed garden for soothing waters. (Mint, lemon balm, lavender, and rosemary often grow in front yards on the West and East Coasts during non-winter months.)

10. Nettles and various tea bags. It's going to feel really good to nuke some water in the hotel or at a friend's house and make tulsi rose tea when you are in a La Quinta Inn in Rohnert Park, California. Nettles will save your ass, give you steady energy and vitamins, and ward off the sick.

11. Roll up a heating pad and take it with you! Plug it in on the Megabus and on the plane, if there are outlets, or in the hotel

or crash space if it's cold. Game changer. You will hurt so much less, and it'll help you not freeze.

12. For the love of God, if you can, give yourself days off in the middle of weeks on the road. Or at least plan to be just fine, ecstatic even, during tour, and then crash like a motherfucker once you get back. Don't plan anything but Netflix, laundry, and water for a couple days after if you can help it. Also, think about how much you can do. For me, two friend visits a day is plenty. Don't let the terrible people who got you off your couch to do art for money schedule you to do three workshops, two meet and greets and a one-person show in one day. Just say no. Also, remember that being outside your comfort zone and having to negotiate public transit and neighborhoods you don't know (or know access info for) is its own stress.

13. Look up where the community acupuncture spots are—there's a big map at *pocacoop.com*—and make an appointment if this works for you. For fifteen dollars, you might get some rest and some relief for what ails you.

14. If you're a YMCA member, make use of the AWAY (Always Welcome at the Y) program. (They have no way of checking if your membership is expired—use that membership you stopped being able to pay for two years ago.) With a membership, you can go to any Y anywhere for free. If they ask, tell them yes, you *do* get free towels at your home Y! Soak in that hot tub!

15. Go ahead and get dip powder, gels, or acrylics before or during tour if you do your nails and this is chemically accessible to you. Your hands are going to look like shit from dragging everything around, and having durable nails will make you feel better and like you are in control of something when you do not control planes showing up late, buses breaking down, etc.

16. Bring powdered, fragrance-free laundry detergent in a ziplock so you can do laundry when everything smells bad. Mostly, no one will have frag-free detergent, especially the laundromat, and you don't want to have to buy a box.

17. Also in a ziplock: coffee and a couple filters, if you drink it, or the tea of your choice.

18. Bring a portable altar—it can be a small candle, an ancestor image, a rock, a place to put water. Keep these in ziplocks. Put them out where you are staying. Makes you feel better.

19. Another access need you may have is to just chill and be alone and soothed. It took me a while to figure this out. But I need time when no one is talking to me and I don't have to be polite and nice to folks I just met or teach a class. I'm really bad at small talk, and I get worse the longer I have to try to do it. Also, I tend to do the kind of performance art that makes everyone want to tell me the most intense shit they've ever been through right after. Which is a blessing but also exhausting. Maybe you're autistic or neurodivergent, maybe you're tired, maybe you're tired of being stared at or of having to figure out the accessible routes through an unfamiliar city. I am in favor of borrowing a totally escapist library book before tour, and having a script in your head to excuse yourself from things—say you need to go rest or have to make a phone call. Motels/hotels are weird, but sometimes they are a haven where you don't have to be "on."

20. I am a cane user, and I have at times brought a cheap folding cane so I don't lose my wooden cane when I'm moving around a lot and my brain fog is up and I start forgetting where everything is. Sometimes I ask for wheelchair assistance, even if I'm feeling more mobile at the beginning of tour, because I know that my pain and fatigue levels are going to skyrocket during tour, and airports are huge and body-wrecking. Wheelchair assistance

means getting to the airport early, so sometimes when I am running late I don't use it, but I do ask for pre-boarding. I used to ask if there was a disability line at the airport, but they no longer exist at many North American airports.

21. Make sure to ask people you're staying with for what you need, sometimes more than once, and be specific. For me, this means: smoke-free rooms, heat, a bed or pullout couch, quiet after eleven p.m., proximity to a place I can store and cook food, a no-stairs setup or an elevator, and a door that shuts. Don't assume that non-crips will get it the first time you say what your needs are, even if they're going "Oh yes" and being real polite. Their "Oh, there's no stairs" is often a flight of stairs.

22. The La Quinta Inn has a hot water dispenser in its breakfast bar! Which means hella nettle tea! If you get a hotel/motel, one with a mini fridge and microwave rocks.

23. Most hotels are able to use fragrance-free cleansers and take the air "freshener" out of the room first if you ask in advance. Get the person booking it to ask for this when they book. They can just say that you have "allergies" or whatever.

24. Bring some cute cotton underwear. You need underwear that can stand up to hours of sitting in buses, trains, cars, and planes. Nylon just helps candida go nuts.

25. Menstruators: the menstrual sponge, cup, or cloth pad is my fav. Cloth pads can be shoved in a ziplock, and they can also be shoved in underwear to absorb twelve hours' worth of blood while you're on Megabus.

26. Finally, this is hard, but I kind of always have in my back pocket the idea that if the worst-case scenario happens—if I get into a severe mental health crisis or get pneumonia—I can cancel. This has been really hard for me as a raised working-class person who often does not have a lot of money (to put it mildly), and as

someone who exists in artist cultures, where there is a culture and reality of scarcity/not enough money/you work for six months for this show that happens one time and pays $100, and if you miss it, your career is over! I'm not saying canceling is easy or always possible, but it has been comforting for me to say to myself, if shit gets really bad, I can reschedule and folks will have to deal. And, especially as I get older, I do and have done this. Maybe there really will never be another show. Maybe there will be. Maybe my capacity is my capacity. Maybe sometimes, or often, I have to push beyond what I can do to survive. Maybe sometimes I can't.

27. When you're booking stuff, try really hard not to do the thing gig organizers will want you to do where they want you to meet students, give a performance, do a workshop, and visit a class all in one day. If that works for you, great. I used to have a hard time saying, "Hey, that's too much for my body," because I thought I'd just get fired, but it turns out sometimes you can ask for this. One or two things a day is enough.

28. Build in access to your requests. Like it's normal. The access you need and the access you might not need. Tell them the gig needs to be in wheelchair-accessible space whether or not you are a chair user. Get ASL booked and have them do it well—promoting to Deaf communities, sending your scripts to the interpreters ahead of time. Build in the idea that it's not just about some weird special diva requests you have. It's about survival and space for all of us.

PART
III

FUCK THE "TRIUMPH OF THE HUMAN SPIRIT"

ON WRITING DIRTY RIVER AS A QUEER, DISABLED, FEMME-OF-COLOR MEMOIR AND THE JOYS OF SAYING FUCK YOU TO TRADITIONAL ABUSE SURVIVOR NARRATIVES

In a week, the memoir *Dirty River: A Queer Femme of Color Dreaming Her Way Home* that I started working on in 2004 hits the shelves of bookstores and e-shopping carts everywhere.[43] It's been ten fucking years of sweating over this book, in DIY writing residencies and the ten-by-ten shack I rented in the back of my QTBIPOC South Berkeley collective house, on Megabuses, and on my phone.

Telling the story of this book coming out is impossible to do without also talking about the politics of publishing survivor narratives and of publishing as a queer femme of color, period. Because there aren't a lot of survivor memoirs, and there aren't a lot of survivor memoirs by queer femmes of color, and there aren't a lot of survivor memoirs that are by queer femmes of color who are crips.

But there are a lot of ideas of what a survivor narrative is. (At least in my head, which, arguably, is stuck in stuff I took in watching *Oprah* and *The Young and the Restless* with my mom in the 1990s.) You know—something terrible and murky happens in a bedroom, there's a lot of DARKNESS, and then the sun comes out, you speak to a nice therapist in a pastel office for six sessions, and then you're

---

43   This essay was first published in September of 2015, on *Third Woman Pulse*'s blog, https://thirdwomanpulse.com, which is offline as of May 2018.

fixed, you marry your husband or get a girlfriend and have a kid, and it's all pastel soft lighting fade out forever. You either do that or you're fucked—you abuse your kids, and you die a horrible death. Those are the two options in the back of folks' heads. Most folks want to go for the Triumph of the Human Spirit one, if you get to pick.

But there are a million survivor stories. As many survivor stories as there are survivors. When I was coming up, as a person, as a writer, reading abuse survivor narratives was one of the things that saved my life—no lie. I am beyond grateful for the writers in the 1980s and '90s who broke the world open writing our stories about the violence we endured. From the zines like *Body Memories* and *Fantastic Fanzine* that I mailed two well-wrapped dollar bills and some soaked stamps to get a copy of to the first time I heard Sapphire perform her poem "Mickey Mouse Was a Scorpio" in 1994 when I was nineteen, from second-wave queer white feminist incest survivor books like Louise Wisechild's *The Obsidian Mirror* and Elly Danica's *Don't: A Woman's Word* to the copy of *Bastard out of Carolina* I shoplifted from the Framingham, MA, Borders, I would be nowhere without this cultural movement—wildly not remembered or included in literary canons—of survivors speaking about and being the experts on our own experiences. We changed the world through writing about how very common sexual assault, childhood sexual abuse, and partner abuse are, and through writing our lived experiences as real and authoritative, in all their weird, perfect, dissociated glory.

But a lot of those books and zines were written twenty years ago. And a lot of the survivor narratives then and since are by white cis women. Queer or punk or working-class white cis women, but white cis women nonetheless. Most of them never mention disability. And that begs the question: What is a survivor narrative by queer people of color, including disabled ones? When June Jordan wrote about her father's abuse in her memoir, *Soldier*, do we think of it as a "survivor narrative"? Why is the only survivor story I can think of that is capital D Disabled by a white femme—Peggy Munson? Do the writings by my Native and/or sex-working friends who do work around missing and murdered Indigenous women count as survivor narratives? Racist tropes of innocent white victims and frenzied Black and brown sexualities and criminality compete so that we as people of color cannot be seen as real survivors—those are pure white cis women off somewhere—and we don't want to show our families and communities for the violent, broken Black and brown things the white world thinks they are anyway. For so many QTBIPOC, surviving violence is just life. We survive so many forms of violence and are resilient, and not. We make it, and we don't, and we make it sideways. Shit is complicated, and shit is weirder than we thought.

So that's what I wanted to do with *Dirty River*. I wanted to write a complex disabled, queer, femme of color survivor memoir. One where my abuse and incest story is not separable from my father's story and mine of moving far away from Sri Lanka through exile and colonization and homophobia. From my mother's story of being a survivor, a crazy genius, a working-class white woman, a polio survivor who never once called herself disabled. I wanted to write a transformative justice story of a violent family whose parents are also survivors, who also taught me things I needed to know to survive. Where the therapist and the cops don't really figure in the story of healing, but homemade Diwalis with other queer Black and brown folks, the queer people of color club night, and being a slutty brown femme on Greyhound with two backpacks and a hoodie sure do.

And—in a way that I couldn't even articulate when I was doing it—I wanted to write survivor stories as disabled stories. *Dirty River* tells part of my story of walking into abuse memories and becoming chronically ill at the same time. But I also wanted to explore my survivor wounds and knowledges—what is known in the biomedical world as complex PTSD—as a disability narrative. I wanted to write about being sick, crazy, deeply tired, brilliant, and dreaming.

In the afterword to Lidia Yuknavitch's memoir *The Chronology of Water*, an interviewer mentions that Yuknavitch never once shows a graphic scene of her father molesting her. She doesn't. When her future husband asks her, "What kind of abuse did your father do?" she says, "Sexual." You see her father's violence in the atmosphere in the house, in the after-party of the damage as she figures her way back to herself through fucking, parenting, kink, queerness, drug use, writing, loss. You see the violence in the tension in the house as her father refuses to let her go to one of the colleges she's gotten scholarships to, in the moment when she grabs a big black suitcase out of the garage and he almost fistfights her for it. She utters the phrase, "It was a suitcase big enough to hold the rage of a girl." But you don't see a clinical depiction of the times he molested her.

Because the other thing I know about survivor narratives—the dynamic of "prove it." Survivors are always and forever asked to show a videotape depicting the most overt, gruesome moments of abuse. Or else it's not real. It's a way the colonial prison-industrial complex invades our ways of thinking about abuse, survivorhood, and what counts as "real." You had something bad happen? Are you sure? Is it really bad? Show us. What's your evidence? How can we trust you, you Black or brown queer or trans sick body? People insist on knowing "what happened" and to them, "what happened" is the most graphic moment of violence possible.

But survivorhood is not just what would be in the police file. Far from it. It is all our stories of every moment we survive. It is all the weirdness and wonder. All the homemade ways we make it. All the ways we are "telling a story that is still being written"—which is a way I heard queer Ashkenazi Jewish witch and organizer Morgan Bassichis describe transformative justice one day when she was leading a workshop at Safetyfest 2011. There are as many survivor stories as there are survivors of abuse and violence. And I have been up all night worrying about what I left out. I have been up all night worried that people will lift this book up as the one queer of color survivor narrative that exists, that everyone should measure themselves by. But it's not. It's one white-mama, brown, AFAB, femme, chronically ill, working-class/mixed-class girl now in their forties story. And it's not about me. I want there to be a million of our books in print, getting to talk to each other.

But because of the publishing industry being what it is, I worry. It's impossible for me to talk about writing *Dirty River* without talking about the politics of the publishing industry for queer people of color writers, in terms of the death of many print institutions and in terms of the intersectional racist weirdness of the publishing-industrial complex. And it's also important for me to talk about my practical, Taurus, how-I-did-it writing process, because there are not enough stories out there by writers of color who do not have trust funds or husbands or full-time jobs saying how we did it.

Working on *Dirty River* over the years has meant watching press after press that was a mainstay of queer, feminist, and independent publishing, like South End, Alyson, Firebrand, Press Gang, or Seal Press, go bust or get eaten by a bigger corporate press. When I graduated from my MFA program at Mills College in 2009, I took two jobs—working as the events coordinator at Modern Times Bookstore, an independent, radical bookstore in the heart of the Mission District, and teaching at UC Berkeley's June Jordan's Poetry for the People program. One paid twelve bucks an hour; the other paid a little more. This was on top of my solo performance work and my work co-running Mangos with Chili, the queer and trans people of color performance tour and collective performing and touring with Sins Invalid, and teaching med students the pelvic exam. (I also managed my chronic illness and got sick and tired as hell because all of this was way too much hustle—I look back and I really wonder why I didn't die.) In my time working at Modern Times, I observed as press after press whose books we sold and booked events for died. The list of places I could query got tighter.

Oh yeah, about grad school—I barely survived undergrad the first time around, but part of the reason I went to grad school was because a few of my writer friends were getting agents and deals in the mid-2000s. I thought, I'll go to grad school, do well, make friends, and maybe one of my teachers will hook me up with her agent, and maybe I'll get a fucking book deal. This is a big part of How It Is Done. I also knew I would never finish a book of prose if I was still co-running the radical Asian/Pacific Islander arts and history program, gigging, freelancing, and working at the eviction prevention hotline. I thought grad school would buy me some time, and I'd be able to teach at the university level once I got the degree.

So I went to grad school. I did okay, even though there was a lot of bullshit and a lot of white women with bleached oak hair named Emily, and even though I had a hard time pretending I was obedient to authority, and I kept taking time off to go on tour with the QTBIPOC performance organization I cofounded. I survived grad school by telling myself that it was something I was doing in my spare time, that Oakland's QTBIPOC arts and performance communities were my real job. I survived because I did learn some stuff from the women of color I studied with, and from fighting to get to learn and teach at Poetry for the People, and because the whole thing made me step up my game, even though a lot of it was bullshit. I made friends with some of the women of color teachers there. One of them did hook me up with her agent. An agent who also represented Michael Ondaatje and a lot of other big-name writers of color. And then the economy tanked in 2008, and the big five media corporations who owned all the major presses weren't taking on much, let alone weirdo alternative queer punk POC memoirs that didn't have a simple happy ending. I didn't get a six-figure book deal, or that agent, or a mainstream press.

I graduated. I kept co-running the QTBIPOC performance collective. I kept reading and performing and throwing events in my femme house in South Berkeley. I got gigs to perform at Oberlin and Wesleyan and Humboldt State. I kept teaching the pelvic exam. I got flown to Australia to speak and got to see my grandparents' graves for the first time. I had cheap rent and was sick and wrote my ass off, and our house got broken into a bunch of times and my computer got stolen. I had lovers and heartbreak and friends and heartbreak. I kept working on *DR* whenever I had time. I got rejected from fancy residencies, and I said fuck it one year and went to Fancyland, the queer rural land project my friends' friend started, and wrote my ass off for two weeks without internet or cell service. Being chronically ill is not the greatest, but you know what? If I were able-bodied and I could hold down a nine-to-five, I probably wouldn't have finished this book that I finished in between part-time gigs working from bed when sick.

The rejections piled up. My rejections ranged from a condescending print letter from an intern saying, "Next time you submit, you should spell-check" (I had. Those weren't spelling errors; that was unconventional POC English) to my friend's small press loving it and then realizing they didn't have enough capacity to publish it well. To the academic feminist press that had given me an award a few years before inviting me to their fancy office for a meeting, where the chief editor who looked like Eileen Myles if she had a husband and a nonfat triple macchiato from Starbucks asked me to explain what transformative justice was, cut me off, and informed me that the experimental novel Muriel Rukeyser had written about the Spanish Civil War that a grad student had found in her files was going to be a bigger hit and sell better than my book, because mine "read more like a performance piece." ("It's luminous," she said about the Muriel Rukeyser.) To the small, nice indie APIA press saying it wasn't experimental enough.

The kind of impostor syndrome you can get sitting there thinking, *I am fucking almost forty years old. My shit is taught in a lot of women's and ethnic studies classrooms. I've cofounded a ton of organizations, performed to sold-out houses all over the country, from Harvard to dyke bars. Things I publish get thousands of hits. There is a huge vibrant queer feminist of color literary, political, and cultural community that I am a part of, that keeps asking when the book is going to come out, that these fools know nothing about. And they still won't offer me a lousy book deal* is huge. As a GIF in my feed said recently, "God, give me a quarter of the confidence of a mediocre white man."

By the time I ripped open the email on my phone in December 2014 and saw that Arsenal Pulp Press—a non-tiny Canadian indie press focused on queer and post/anti-colonial literature, with a queer Asian editor, weren't just willing, they were excited to publish *Dirty River,* I had resigned myself. They were it—the only press left. If they didn't say yes, I was going to go on Indiegogo and raise money to self-publish. Because Nia King had done that with *Queer & Trans Artists of Color: Stories of Some of Our Lives,* and that book is a QTBIPOC bestseller. Because there wasn't going to be another option. But part of me still really wanted a press. Because it's harder to get your self-published work into libraries and on reading lists and submitted to awards. And I have always wanted my books to be work that's possible for libraries to order, so broke folks can read it for free.

And look—I am oppressed, but I am well aware that I have certain privileges on my side. I am a US citizen with an MFA and light skin, and I am not impacted by transmisogyny. Writers without those privileges face even more struggles to get published.

I don't want to end on a sad note. And I don't have to. Because queer Black and brown writers from Ryka Aoki de la Cruz to Meliza Bañales, from Kai-Cheng Thom to Alexis Pauline Gumbs keep figuring out how to get our shit out there in the world. From the trans-women-of-color-led Biyuti Press's works to Meliza's novel *Life Is Wonderful, People Are Terrific,* we keep defying all odds and publishing not-small books at small presses that have a big impact, as our people always have. Those feminist and queer and POC small presses of the 1970s and '80s were created in basements. Kitchen Table Press was literally created at a kitchen table. We always create the technology, from lipstick to Tumblr, we need to survive. And that includes publishing our writing, on our own terms, for the people who want and need to read it.

SUICIDAL IDEATION 2.0

QUEER COMMUNITY LEADERSHIP, AND STAYING ALIVE ANYWAY

For my beloved dead, for Kyle and Wendy, and for all of us still here

I've come to hate it when folks start texting me with cryptic messages saying, *Did you know so-and-so?*

For the past two years, each summer, my beloved community in Toronto has lost someone because they killed themselves. This year, it was Kyle Scanlon.[44]

And no, I didn't really know him—not well—but I knew of him. Kyle was one of the first trans guys I knew, who came out in Toronto's queer community in the late 1990s. After he passed, many, many trans folks remembered how Kyle had come to their workplace or school and told his story, how he was the first other trans person they'd met. How his story and presence helped them name themselves as trans and do what they needed to do to affirm the gender spirit that made them feel alive. Kyle was one of the first workers at Meal Trans, the free dinner program at the 519 (Toronto's queer community center) for broke trans folks. He won awards and did trainings. He was one of those queer/trans community-bred and -based leaders everybody thanks, leans on, asks for favors, and is grateful for.

And he killed himself.

---

44 This piece was written in summer 2012. I've kept the original wording.

After he died, there were the blog posts saying we had to love each other harder and do better. There were the memorial posts that listed all the distress center hotlines for the province. There were the postings of his memorial articles from the queer biweekly paper on Facebook and everyone's memories. It's what we do. And it so wasn't enough.

Moments like this are grief and crash. And they're also—maybe—an invitation to go deeper. To be real about suicide. I mean really really for real for real—about shit that people don't want to go there about or want to boil down into a simple narrative of *Don't do it; you have something to live for! Call 911!* Even the narratives we have that suicide is the colonizer, is the white supremacist capitalist colonialist ableist patriarchy whispering that we should just take ourselves off the planet—that narrative has stopped me from reaching for my Ativan and bourbon or cutting when I didn't want to. But they're also not enough.

I was in Toronto the week after Kyle died, with my family. Everyone was hurting. Some of us at Femme Heartshare Circle were talking about it. About how Wendy Babcock, an amazing street sex worker activist, mama, and law student, had died of an overdose last year, and how folks weren't sure whether it was intentional—and how Wendy's family had used her history of struggling with mental health to discredit her courage in talking about the abuse from them she'd survived.

One of my friends said, "What should we do? Should we have regular red flag check-ins with each other, the way we do about relationships? Should I go up to you and ask, 'Have you been thinking about killing yourself lately?'" And I thought, *If anyone came at me saying, HAVE YOU THOUGHT ABOUT KILLING YOURSELF LATELY?, I'd automatically lie and say, hell no.* The way I have to every single doctor, social worker, and most therapists in my life. Like any smart crazy, I don't want anything I can prevent on my permanent record, and I definitely don't want Danger to Self or Others. I've been fighting this my whole life, and I've seen the oppression and hardness that label can mean to folks.

But if you normalized it. Because it is normal. This secret. That so many of us wrestle with suicidality. Then maybe, maybe, just maybe I'd tell you where I was at.

And maybe we could map the terrain of those ideation places better.

I don't know why Kyle killed himself. But his death, and the regular punctuation of queer and trans suicides in our forties, makes me think. We have narratives that focus on how hard it is not to die when we are young and queer, trans, or Two Spirit. And those are very necessary. But maybe we should also be getting real about what it takes to keep queer and gender-variant and Two-Spirit adults alive too.

As a queer or trans or Two-Spirit adult, we live within narratives that say that if you just live to grow up, it gets better (Dan Savage is an asshole caveat aside).

But: What if it gets better and transforms more than you ever expected, but there are also times when it's still crazy, hurts so bad? Maybe hurts worse because it did get better, it got so much better, and also, the struggle did not stop? You ended up sleeping in the back of your station wagon on a mattress pad. Your book went out of print. Your mama died. You were still crazy after all that cum and all those tears. And no one prepared you for a life narrative where maybe struggle and therapy and herbs and miracles healed the pain, but the pain didn't go all the way away. Maybe, as you survived and succeeded, it just got more complex.

Take me. I know it because I am also one of those community leaders. I am one of those community leaders who at thirty-seven still sometimes feels so low. My life did get better. I am not the same tortured, disassociated girl I was. I look good. I'm happy. I'm not strangled by self-hatred in the every-single-second-of-every-day way my eighteen-year-old brain knew. I have had the gay sex and art and travel and books and home and all of it. My brain and my spirit and my life and my relationship to trauma have changed, deeply. And I still have suicidal ideation on the regular.

I've had suicidal ideation (where you have repeating thoughts of *I should just kill myself*) since I was at least twelve years old. From when I was about twelve to twenty-one, I had periods of months or years when I had to seriously fight suicidality. When I was twenty-two, I got away from my abusive family, left the country, made my small, quiet, safe room, and started healing hard-core from the shit I'd grown up in.

Since the therapy and the small, quiet, safe room and the poetry and the dancing and the friends and the lovers and the herbs and the words, since shit stopped being as nuclear fucked up as my childhood was, I don't really really wanna kill myself anymore. I don't have a plan. I don't actively want to do it. I love my life. I am blessed. I am joyful. I am happy. But at times—at times of deep grief, or deep stress, or sometimes even times that aren't even that fucking deep—sometimes, I sit for hours, my wrists on fire with the desire to cut.

I won the Lambda Literary Award this year, and it was one of the best feelings of my life. And three days later, for no damn reason and every damn reason, I left therapy and felt my mood crashing. I tried to drive to a friend's birthday party, but the directions were complicated and I circled five times before giving up and driving home. I crawled into bed at three p.m. and found myself staring at the pillbox on my dresser, thinking, *I've got five Ativan and a bottle of good bourbon. Is that enough?*

And I thought, *Whoa.* And I thought, *I am thirty-seven and I just won the Lambda Award. I can't tell people I want to kill myself. On my Facebook status update.*

I slept. I texted a lover I'd had the sweetest access intimacy with to ask about Wellbutrin. I called friends. I called my witch naturopath in Toronto, who saw me on Skype for twenty bucks and asked me, "What does the depression feel like?" I told her it felt like a slow, soft river, that it was good I had a lot of great things in my life, but even when I was in them right then, I couldn't really feel them. And when things did get bad, the direct line to *Ishouldjustkillmyself* was well marked. I talked to my somatic therapist about CBT, and I started taking 5-HTP, a serotonin precursor.

We believe that working for justice and healing, creating art, and being badasses on our own terms will be part of what heals our hurt. And it is. But our communities also put enormous pressure on the community-based queer leaders we look to, and are. The leadership paradigm that exists within queer and trans social justice communities is still that of the movement/activist star. As much as we may critique it, we don't quite have another one yet. We have complicated feelings about leaders. We need role models. We want to celebrate folks who are talented organizers and artists. And we also don't know how to practice horizontal leadership. We lift people up and pedestalize them—expect them to be perfect and have all the answers. We tear them down, murder folks who look like and unlike us when we fuck up, make mistakes, aren't able to be always on call, or just politically disagree. We don't know how to let people be both gifted and imperfect. And when we are those people, going from being a nobody to being a movement star, well, it doesn't leave a lot of room for complexity. Or to feel comfortable being honest about wanting to die when so many people are looking to you for a reason to live.

And our communities are still struggling to know how to care for each other well. For real. For the long term. Without shame, when it doesn't get fixed perfectly the first time.

When I've wanted to kill myself—when it's hit strong and knocked me to my knees familiar—there's this thing. It's felt like, in that moment, I can feel all the ways I really have been without agency in my life.

And in that moment of feeling the deep grief and sadness over the impact of oppression, killing myself has felt like one clear way I can have agency. I can have total control. I can't control the WSCCAP. But I can go to the stars.

And it hits fast. With Wendy, with Kyle, and with other folks who've killed themselves in my communities, it's not uncommon for folks to say, I just saw them the other day. They were happy. They were fine. And they might've been. They might've been holding a lot of hard shit they didn't know how to talk about. And they might've gone from wonderful to deeply despairing fast—and not had room or words to talk about that, or felt deeply ashamed of freaking out, yet again.

What does it mean for those of us who made things better, who are shaped in the shape of *I will come through for you,* who have organized and created curriculums and built programs and won awards and fought and mentored and let folks crash on our couches—what happens when we are, again, the crazy, hurting, deeply sad inside places? That are so different from the ones maybe so many outsiders know?

When sometimes we ask for help on Facebook and miracles come through, and sometimes we do and our GoFundMe falls flat? When we are afraid that we were hurting six months ago, and we're hurting now, and what is the tipping point when people start thinking, *There they go again, they're always freaking out.*

I think about the deep and complicated stigma of crazy—the reality that even in radical communities where sometimes we are better about loving people who are "too much," we also know the fear of crazy. The reality of community that is love but also just likes to kick it and be casual. Or the roommate wanted ad for the collective house I once looked at that said, *We're cool with you having mental or physical health concerns as long as you take care of them on your own and don't bring that shit into the house.* I think about how the crazy take care of the crazy when no one else will, and when we're not in crisis ourselves, sometimes we want a break.

We don't want platitudes or uplift or people telling us we're loved. I mean, tell me. But I know I'm loved. Sometimes hearing that helps. Sometimes I am still deeply, deeply sad anyway. I don't have the answers, but I am interested in collectively creating them. I am interested in all of us who dance with dying talking about all the different and real things that suicide can mean to us. All the things that allow us to stay here. And more than that, I am interested in creating models of happy mostly queer and trans adulthood where we can be leaders and still be vulnerable, where we can be open that it's not happily ever after. Life models that encompass falling apart and reforming not as a failure but as a life pathway. Ones punctuated with whirlwinds and whirlpools, that Coatlicue/Kali/Oya energy that dismembers. And gifts.

SO MUCH TIME SPENT IN BED

A LETTER TO GLORIA ANZALDÚA ON CHRONIC
ILLNESS, COATLICUE, AND CREATIVITY

ANOTHER FIBROMYALGIC QUEER BROWN GIRL MORNING

Dear Gloria,

Dawn. Sunrise floats through the window slats of my shack, the little EI-safer house in the back of the queer collective house I inhabit. Some days, I will rise now. Some days, I will hit the snooze button for three hours. I will turn over and over in my big bed. I will shift. I will get up oh, so slowly. How damp is it out, how bad is my pain, how shaky is my balance and my cognitive ability today? Yet another fibro morning. Dawn creeps past my eyelids and I shove her away. Not yet! My fatigue—the deep fatigue of chronic illness, untouched by days and weeks of good sleep, not the fatigue of a night staying up too late—has not been touched today. I turn over and down. I drift back to sleep.

My life is bookended by library books, vibrator, and baths. Something more than simple self-care, and something other than a life of a lazy, privileged girl. It is a crip life, a chronically ill life. It is a life of dreamtime.

I am a chronically ill, disabled writer. I am a queer woman of color writer. I have a shelf full of anthologies with my words in them. I have been able to pursue the path of red and black ink.

I am a queer femme of color writer. I am a chronically ill femme.

My entire adult life has been marked by illness. It's hard for me to tell when the pain, butterfly balance, fatigue, and immune transparency I name as fibromyalgia really started. A childhood filled with abuse, terror, and a need to sleep as much as possible bleeds into chronically tired yet overachieving college years, bleeds into the early twenties when I walked back into my incest memories, got sick, and spent a lot of time on my futon, struggling with fatigue, pain, and shakiness.

Fibromyalgia is the name I choose for the constellation of repeating cycles of fatigue, muscle pain that does not have an organic source, immune system meltdowns, shakiness, balance problems, and cognitive delay that hit me when I am stressed or doused with chemicals. Yoga, a regular bedtime, flextime, herbs, quitting smoking, kale and protein and quinoa all helped, but there is no cure for this body. This is my body. This syndrome is new/old and ongoing, unfolding. It changes as we find new ways to think about trauma, our bodies, embodiment, environmental racism, and sickness.

Chronic illness sucks. But, oh, there is the secret bliss of bed! Chronic illness may not have made me a writer, but it illuminates my writing life. I can't work a 9-to-5—the times I tried left me winded in bed after three days—but bed time means lots of dreamtime. Sometimes it's low-quality dreamtime—dreamtime where I am zonked on half a Soma, watching internet TV, using my vibrator, and alternating soaking in hot baths with lying on a big ice pack to manage my pain. But whether it is high- or low-quality dreamtime, being a sick femme means I have more dreamtime than most 9-to-5 or movement organizers could ever dream of!

It is so difficult to write both what sucks about disability—the pain, the oppression, the impairment—and the joy of this body at the same time. The joy of this body comes from crip community and interdependence, but most of all, of the hard beauty of this life, built around all the time I must spend resting. The bed is the nepantla place of opening.

Capitalism says that disabled, tired bodies that spend too much time in bed are useless. Anyone who cannot labor to create wealth for owners is useless. People are valued only for the wealth they labor to build for capitalism; crips are useless to capitalism. That's why social programs are cut, why Hitler referred to us as "useless eaters"—we often are not able to be fast, assembly-line workers who produce wealth for someone else.

I am a chronically ill queer of color artist, and so much of my time is spent in bed. I joke that my bed, heaped with cushions, is my office, my world headquarters. My life is arranged around my bed. There is good art to look at, a window, my vibrator plugged in, a stack of books within easy reach.

I lie in it thinking of all my other crip poet friends who spend most of their days in bed too. Draped in pillows, red and plum sheets, surrounded by good art to look at, curtained by plum sari fabric. This is my place of power, the fulcrum, the place everything emerges from.

I dream here. I write here.

What I know is that Gloria Anzaldúa and I meet in bed. Not like you think. Maybe like you think. Gloria and I meet in bed. It's sexy. And it's just life. Gloria and I meet in bed, in the chronically ill sickbed heaped with pillows where we both spend so much time.

Gloria, we meet in bed. You never said you were disabled, that I can find—every inch of evidence you left resisted that label. But whatever you felt about that world, this is where you dreamed and lived too. This place of bodily difference, a tired body that comes in pain and suffering, that allows us to work part-time weird jobs, to rest, to fly.

1938: Gloria is born in Hargill, Texas. At three months, her mother sees tiny pink dots of menstrual blood on her diaper and freaks the fuck out. The doctor says, "Don't worry, she's a throwback to the eskimo—eskimo girls get their periods early." Is she intersex? Would she call herself that now? She calls herself *jota, mita y mita,* half and half, the way lesbians are called in South Texas. Her breasts develop at eight years old; there is a secret, a folded rag pinned to her underwear, in grade school, her breasts bound down tight with bandages by her mother. "Keep your legs shut, Prieta."[45] In her twenties and thirties, fibroids and 104-degree fevers rock her body monthly. In her forties, she develops diabetes. During the week of May 15, 2004, Gloria Evangelista Anzaldúa transitions to the ancestors/dies of complications related to diabetes. She is sixty-one. She is marked by physical difference all her life, from the blue spot on her butt at birth, the mark of African blood and the ability to see beyond, to pain, the need for rest.

1979: Gloria decides to devote her life to writing, takes a series of part-time lecturer and writer-in-residence jobs to buy as much time to write as possible.

1991: Gloria wins an NEA grant, uses it to buy a house in Santa Cruz by her beloved ocean, Yemaya, so she can visit it daily.

A quote from "Speaking in Tongues: A Letter to 3rd World Women Writers": "It is dark and damp and has been raining all day. I love days like this. As I lie in bed I am able to delve inward. Perhaps today I will write from the deep core."

She writes while other people sleep. She writes of getting up, sitting down, looking for, and always, the writing.[46] The path of red and black ink.

Gloria, the written record I have access to is often silent about how sick you were, how much those knifelike fibroid pains, those energy drops from diabetes that stole your life early, affected your life. But on the record is how you stole dreamtime. Stole time to write and dream. You stayed up all night, slept all day. You joked about how you would do anything, anything to avoid the writing—clean house, make nopalitos, take a bath, burn candles. But you knew the writing was always there,

---

45   This passage contains quotes and paraphrasings from Gloria Anzaldúa, "La Prieta," in *This Bridge Called My Back: Writings by Radical Women of Color*, edited by Cherríe Moraga and Gloria Anzaldúa (Boston: Kitchen Table/Women of Color Press, 1984), 221.

46   Gloria Anzaldúa, "Speaking in Tongues: A Letter to 3rd World Women Writers," in *This Bridge Called My Back*, 169.

waiting, your constant lover and companion. The toad inside that makes poems open to you. You chose writing over lovers, over others. You wrote of being a bridge, drawbridge, or island—identifying finally as a sandbar, a natural formation that could be connected or isolated as the tides turned. Like the tides of our bodies—our sick, in pain, in less pain bodies that resist a boxed-in life that an ableist world demands.

Queer people of color never say we are disabled if we have any choice about it. We come from families who believe in being tough, in sucking it up. We do not want any more identities than we already have to wrestle with. Our bodies already seen as tough, monster, angry, seductive, incompetent. How can we admit weakness, vulnerability, interdependence and still keep our jobs, our perch on the "thin edge of barbwire" we live on? Why would we join crips who are all white in the mainstream rights movement?

How do we claim this body broken beautiful as not a liability but a gift? To know that interdependence is what has saved us time and time again—as queers and trans people, people of color, women, broke folks. How my lovers and friends help each other survive—passing twenty dollars back and forth across the movement, driving me to get groceries when I can't make it down the stairs.

How do we say that my hurting body in bed sucks and is also a beautiful ability to write for hours because I can't hold down a 9-to-5 even if I wanted to?

And part of the beauty is our access to dream time. Time for the stories to grow. Time that is not logical, rational, clock time, punch-the-clock time. At thirty-five, I am surrounded by people who say, "How do you have time to write those poems and stories, cocreate those projects? How are you so productive?" I am so productive because when my gut tells me to take a day off, I do. I lie, say I have a family emergency. When I was a kid I knew that I was supposed to grow up and work a 9-to-5 job, but I didn't ever understand quite how it would happen. I follow the words out my belly. I give in to the bed, to the dreams, to the long, long sleeps and times curled up, the words curl close to me because of them.

How can I say that being chronically ill is a gift? That maybe I would not have become a writer if I had not been too sick and tired to work? That I had to figure something else out? My illness opens the door to write in the nepantla place. Takes me to the path of red and black ink, to where the stories go.

In one of the few scholarly pieces that name Anzaldúa as disabled, AnaLouise Keating writes, "Although Anzaldúa had been living with diabetes for over a decade, many of her readers were unaware of the disease's ongoing, debilitating effects on her life. Even those of us who knew her well were shocked by her sudden death. As Kit Quan, one of Anzaldúa's oldest friends and writing comadres explains, 'Gloria always told me that she was going to stick around for 20 more years. She struggled with diabetes and all its complications daily ... but she was so well read on the disease ... and worked so hard at managing her blood sugars that I believed we still had more time.'"[47]

If I say all this story, maybe no one will be surprised at my death. Maybe someone will know when I get really sick. Maybe I will have enough time. Maybe my sick, dreaming, flying, writing body will have enough people around it who recognize that place for its strength and weakness too. But when I roll over onto my pink T-shirt fabric sheets on another disabled woman of color artist day, feeling the bliss of the cotton on my sore body, when I sleep late and stay up late typing, I feel your body brushing against me. We brush our sick bodies that hurt and also fly. Our sickness a road out from the 9-to-5, trading labor for cash life. Our bodies can't work like that, so they dream instead. Steal time for dreams, poetry, world changing, on that thin edge of barbwire. We dream a way

---

47   AnaLouise Keating, "Introduction: Shifting Worlds, una Entrada," in *EntreMundos/ Among Worlds: New Perspectives on Gloria Anzaldúa*, edited by AnaLouise Keating (London: Palgrave Macmillan, 2005), 9.

through the teeth of the dragon of whitecapitalistpatriarchal amerika. Turn over, write another line. Poems flying in our teeth.

"*Caminante, no hay puentes, se hace puentes al andar.*" Voyager, there are no bridges, one builds them as one walks.

PRINCE, CHRONIC PAIN, AND LIVING TO GET OLD

The reports started to trickle in. They were conflicting, but they still painted a picture: Prince lived with chronic pain for years from all that dancing in high heels and jumping off stages. His knees hurt so bad all the time. He'd had a hip replacement, or he'd needed a hip replacement, but his religion didn't allow him to do it. Prince had flu that turned into walking pneumonia, for three weeks of tour, and he canceled some shows but not others, and he was on a lot of planes. In an *Entertainment Tonight* article that came out right after his passing in 2016, his longtime friend and collaborator Sheila E. said, "He was in pain all the time. But he was a performer."[48]

I had walking pneumonia last week, my second pneumonia this year. I still have it as I am writing this. And right after I went to urgent care with shortness of breath and got the diagnosis, after telling my partner I was just fine for days, I was thinking about still getting on a plane to LA, with pneumonia on three days of antibiotics because the doctor said it should be just fine. I listened to my body, but I had to fight to do so. My sick and disabled friends had to say NO when I asked if maybe, possibly it was okay for me to fly; after all, it was just a mild pneumonia and just a little flight. When I conceded that they were right, I negotiated with the folks offering me the gig while sitting in a chair in the Rite Aid pharmacy waiting area, waiting for my antibiotics to be filled, asking if they'd be open to me doing the

---

48   Antoinette Bueno, "EXCLUSIVE: Sheila E. on Prince: 'He Was in Pain All the Time, but He Was a Performer,'" *ET Online*, April 22, 2016.

talk on Skype so I could be at home, not on a plane and a shuttle and a hotel. And I still wished I could be there in person. I love access, I am grateful for Skype, and I know what it means to still want to be there, in the flesh.

I am very clear I am nowhere near Prince's level of fame, talent, or world domination, his place in the world and what he meant to folks. But I am a writer who goes on tour, and his death made me think about some things about illness, pain, and being a performer.

So here's what I've got: to me, it feels like performance, writing, and art can last forever in the minds of those who witness it. And it's also fragile and easily forgotten, especially if you are a queer/trans artist of color, a disabled queer/trans artists of color, an artist coming from being working class or poor, a rural artist, or all of the above. I often feel like if I stop, everyone will forget about me in five minutes. And this doesn't come from nowhere. It comes from seeing Black and brown queer artists I consider my friends and comrades and also mentors, people a little older than me, people I looked up to and still do, who shared their skills of how to book a show, how to write a grant, how to believe in yourself as a QTBIPOC artist. Artists who maybe hit a rough patch where the thing called life was happening a little more than usual, or just changed the kind of work they were doing or how much they were doing it, and now folks a little younger than me say, "Who?" when their names come up. The laws of perpetual performance motion, as I've experienced them, dictate that you've gotta just keep saying yes to people who want you to come perform or write or do something, because if you say no, the wheels will stop and it's all over. Maybe (probably) this feels different to folks who are artists who have access to wealth or a trust fund. But for most of the rest of us, it feels really different; the model we are taught is to never stop.

I know the feeling of panic when the three gigs I was counting on for fall 2014 all fell through and I was (really) short on money and scared. I know the hustle, the scramble to get money together, to email and follow up. I know all the ways we are superheroes, what it feels like to perform right after puking or having a panic attack and making it shine anyway. I know the ups and downs, and the waiting for the check to show up. I know the feeling of loving what you do and having adrenaline carry you. I know the feeling of post-tour crash after you are home safe in your bed and your body knows it is safe to finally get sick, and you get sick and sick and sick. I know the feeling of fighting to stay relevant and known—not because you want to be famous, but because if people know your work, you'll get work, and your work might reach folks. If not, you won't, and it won't. I know the feeling of loving tour, of feeling blessed to be able to travel around and do what you love for folks. And I know the feeling that you are lucky to be able to do your work and you just have to keep going and going because this is not a 9-to-5 job, so all of this is worth it, right?

As a particular kind of disabled person who for years was broke and sick and unable to leave my neighborhood much, let alone the city, touring was both something other working-class artists explained to me as a way of making a living that could work with the peaks and crashes of a chronically ill body who had fatigue weeks and energy weeks, where you could make a chunk of money and then live frugally off it when you were sick or tired. And something that felt like, and is, an immense privilege that many people don't get to do—for lots of reasons, including that I am a walkie, and it's easier for me to get on buses and trains and planes than many of my friends and comrades who use adaptive devices that public transportation is too ableist to accommodate. I also often default to feeling like no matter how hard things are, I don't have my mom's life—I am not a working-class woman in a shitty marriage with two jobs, rarely leaving her rust belt city, let alone flying all across the country. I am lucky as hell. I got no reason to complain.

And there is truth to all of that. What is also true is all the days you work sick and in pain. All the invisibilized labor you do to lie down before and after, to take pain meds and stretch and carry traditional Chinese medicine tea pills with you to ward off or mitigate the sick, to take care of the sick and pain that happens on the road and after the road. The inner and outer voices and archetypes common in performance culture that say you are so lucky to do what you do, that the show must go on, that you power through illness, that canceling means you're a diva or "unreliable" or weak, that to be open about illness means people will think twice about booking you and think you are no longer at the peak of your career.

What is true for me, post forty, is realizing that the ways I was able to push myself, even as a chronically ill artist, to take red eyes and buses and long, long travel days to shows and workshops and gigs in my thirties, are less possible in my forties.

Many folks I know increasingly talk a lot about sustainability, but I know few who have actually figured out how to do it all the way. That's not our fault—it's ableist capitalism's. We are all trying to survive the best we can, and there are few working artist workshops, fewer working disabled artist workshops, and a reality that it certainly feels like not everyone can make any kind of living as an artist. We are used to doing a lot on a little as a working-class, QTBIPOC artist model of our strengths. We don't have a model of touring that includes disability and illness, canceling and rescheduling, that seems like something other than a luxury, or even possible. This often comes from a place of being cash poor, but it's also true that artists with access to more money don't feel like it's possible to cancel or slow down either.

When Sins Invalid bumped our big October 2010 show to April 2011 after a collective member had three big health issues come up, it was both unprecedented—something no one in performance worlds I know had seen done—and something we did deliberately did as a disability justice collective committed to leaving no one behind and centering our bodies as they were.[49] I hope it's made other groups start to dream how to make performances happen where canceling or rescheduling isn't an unforeseen disaster or an impossibility but something we can plan for.

I don't have a magical solution. But I know that as I write this, I am forty-one, a performer and writer, on my second pneumonia in two months, watching a lot of our beloved artists—Prince so much among them but also Aiyyana Maracle, Mohawk Trans Elder, writer, and performance artist—who meant so much to me and so many folks in communities I am a part of, who just passed from liver cancer as I finished this piece—become ancestors in their forties and fifties and sixties. And I am committed to figuring out together how we can remake performance culture's expectations and figure out our own disabled and chronically ill performance ideas that allow our bodyminds to thrive. I want us to live to get old.

---

49   You can learn more about this decision at "Sins Invalid Performance Update," *Sins Invalid*, September 9, 2010, http://sinsinvalid.org/blog/sins-invalid-performance-update and "Sins Says Thanks," *Sins Invalid*, December 23, 2010, http://sinsinvalid.org/blog/sins-says-thanks.

TWO OR THREE THINGS I KNOW FOR SURE ABOUT FEMMES AND SUICIDE

A LOVE LETTER

Let our wounds scar in good-looking ways.
—Erica Freas

In the day-to-day femme functions as a dare, a longing,
and a political decision about how to move in the world
... Femme smiles while looking at me dead in the eye
saying: I dare you to join me in doing all we can to get
free and get to that other world we have one foot in,
while leaving no parts of our beautiful selves behind.
—Jess St. Louis[50]

Sometimes, I think of the past three years as "the femme suicide years."

In March 2015, I was getting off a plane at JFK after INCITE!'s Color of Violence 4 conference when I looked down at my phone and found out Taueret Davis, Black fat femme burlesque artist, sexual health educator, writer, and community organizer, had taken her life.

Ten months later, I woke up to a text that said, *call me before you go on FB*. I called: the femme on the other end of the line told me about

---

50   From the essay "Femme Taught Me the Difference between Staying Alive and Choosing Aliveness: And Other Thoughts on Desire, Organizing, and Transformation," Medium, June 29, 2017, https://medium.com/@stlouis_j/femme-taught-me-the-difference-between-staying-alive-and-choosing-aliveness-and-other-thoughts-on-675509ffb4ad, accessed November 14, 2018.

the suicide of white, Appalachian, HIV-positive, trans femme writer, theater artist, musician, and hairstylist Bryn Kelly.

The summer after that, Jerika Bolen, a fourteen-year-old Black, queer, disabled femme person with spinal muscular atrophy 2, announced her planned suicide, saying, "I'm going to be free." Bolen gained mainstream media attention for her requested death when she started an Indiegogo to raise money for "Jerika's Last Dance" prom in the month before she would go into hospice and ask them to shut off her ventilator, actions the media named as "brave" and "inspirational." She said that she didn't have a future, that she of course wouldn't be able to dance or date or love, so she was choosing to die, and her announcement of her planned public suicide was cheered on by her white adoptive family and mostly white rural farming community of Appleton, Wisconsin.

As Diane Coleman of the disability activist group Not Dead Yet wrote, "SMA Type II is not a condition that is typically fatal in children and teens. In fact, while some people with SMA die in younger adulthood due to respiratory complications, people with SMA Type II often live into their 60s and beyond. Certainly, SMA would not result in the death of a fourteen-year-old who is receiving appropriate medical care."[51] She used a ventilator as an everyday piece of adaptive technology. Many disabled folks I knew, including myself, were wracked with grief and pain at the spectacle of white, able-bodied family cheering on her death; in their lack of valuing of her life, we saw the ways our own lives weren't seen as valuable or brave. Some wrote Jerika, telling her that they had lives and lovers and jobs and pleasure and dancing, that we wanted her to know her disability did not have to mean a death sentence, and were jeered at by her family community. Why were we sticking our noses into it? It didn't have anything to do with us. It was a "private matter"—even

---

51 Diane Coleman, "Statement on Mourning the Death of Jerika Bolen," *Not Dead Yet*, September 23, 2016, http://notdeadyet.org/2016/09/statement-on-mourning-the-death-of-jerika-bolen.html, accessed July 17, 2018.

though it was in the *Washington Post*.[52] Like many disabled people considering suicide, Jerika was told she was brave to think about dying, not that fighting for the systemic supports that would let her live well would be a brave thing to do. Her announcement of her planned death hovered over our rehearsals for Sins Invalid's 2016 show *Birthing, Dying, Becoming Crip Wisdom*, which, ironically, was a show about just those issues—disabled wisdom, becoming disabled elders, what it meant to live to get old. She died while we were in rehearsal.

Three weeks after Jerika's death, I was on Stinson Beach during Sins tech week with a friend who was struggling when I got the *Don't tell anyone yet, but I wanted you to know before it hit Facebook* text from a friend saying white Southern femme photographer Amanda "Arkansassy" Harris had killed herself. Amanda passed just weeks after her *Femme Space*[53] project, a photography exhibit of femmes taking up space in places where we had been marginalized, had closed after an acclaimed run at San Francisco's National Queer Arts Festival and Harris was named one of KQED's Bay Area Women to Watch.

2016 seemed to be a year where the ancestors were being called home rapidly, maybe to get the fuck out when they still could to avoid the Trump hell that was coming, or maybe to help guide us. Maybe both. This circle of femme death upon death felt like something else.

---

52   For a mainstream media coverage of Bolen's death, see Rachel Premack, "'I'm Going to Be Free': Terminally Ill Wisconsin Teen Schedules Her Death and One 'Last Dance'" *Washington Post*, July 21, 2016, https://www.washingtonpost.com/news/morning-mix/wp/2016/07/21/one-last-dance-for-this-wisconsin-teen-who-has-scheduled-her-own-death/, accessed June 19, 2018. For a disabled analysis, see Diane Coleman, "Statement on Mourning the Death of Jerika Bolen," *Not Dead Yet*, September 23, 2016, http://notdeadyet.org/2016/09/statement-on-mourning-the-death-of-jerika-bolen.html, accessed June 19, 2018.

53   For media coverage of *Femme Space* and some photos, visit Amanda Arkansassy Harris, "Femmes to the Front: Portraits of Queer Femme Identity, an Excerpt from *Femme Space* by Amanda Arkansassy Harris," *East Bay Express*, August 30, 2016, https://www.eastbayexpress.com/oakland/femmes-to-the-front-portraits-of-queer-femme-identity/Content?oid=4955846, accessed June 19, 2018.

Like tall trees, falling. Like losing the ones we needed the most when we needed them the most.

Femme suicide isn't new—we have lost femmes before, like Mark Aguhar, and we've lost femmes since and will again. But that doesn't make it easier. And living through losing five people in three years wasn't easy. All these suicides hit femme and queer communities hard and have prompted mourning, despair, and many community conversations about femmes and suicidality.

After the past three years of public femme suicides, I have been waiting for the moment when I might write something that would be useful. After many drafts, here it is. This is a love letter to all femmes who have taken our lives, to all of us who struggle daily, silently and screaming, with suicidality, and to all of us for the emotional labor we do to help support loved ones dancing with wanting to die. I've been a femme who's wanted to die sometimes for most of my life, and I've loved suicidal femmes and queers for just as long. This is where the story starts.

Queer femme suicide is not a sidenote to the struggle. Queer femme suicide wends its way through every moment of my disabled-queer-femme-of-color-from-a-rust-belt-town political life. My first struggle as a young, utterly fucked, mixed, brown, femme survivor was to stay alive. Continuing to study my suicide science, my reasons to live, to chart the ebb and flow within my deep sadness and my intrusive thoughts, the trauma bombs that go off and nudge me towards death as a best practice and the forces that defuse them, to mine the minerals from them and turn them into the blast furnace that fuels my life is a lifelong marathon.

So here are some things I know sort of for sure about femmes and suicide:

Being perceived as too much can kill you. Femmes are stereotyped across the board as "too much": too loud, too crazy, too emotional, too demanding, too many accessories. "High maintenance," "needy," "hysterical" are curse words. Black and brown femmes, trans femmes, and disabled femmes are stereotyped even more as "too much"—automatically seen as angry, crazy, harsh, hysterical. So when a femme is actually feeling "too much"—sitting with overwhelming feelings of rage and despair and panic—it can feel overwhelmingly hard to reach out and expect that your crazy or your despair won't be too much for the community and loved ones to hold.

"Just call me!" isn't enough. After Amanda's death, many well-meaning people made public announcements urging friends and loved ones to call if they were thinking about dying. Although this is a good first step and an absolutely loving, well-meaning offer, I don't think it's anywhere near enough. Saying, "Please just call me if you feel desperate" is useless if we are not also actively unpacking how ableism makes it damn hard and unsafe to be crazy in public. Most of us have learned damn well that crazy femmes are not loved or respected in queer community or the world—that we're only loved when we're competent, together, and holding it down. For those of us oppression automatically labels as "crazy"—many trans femmes and disabled femmes, for starters—this is doubly true. Add to that intense shame about being "a burden," worry about burning out friends we have, and intense societal expectations that femmes are caregivers of emotional labor without ceasing 24-7, never the ones who get to receive (then you'd just be "needy," right?), and it's no wonder that some of us decide we're doing our people a favor by dying rather than asking. "Ableism" is a word many folks don't know or use in their daily lives. But ableism is what lies within this hatred of femme trauma need, the lit match to the fuse that can lead to femme death.

Femme worship can kill you if you are not also loved in your mess. After these femme suicides, I saw masculine people write testimonials exposing how much they loved (or more often "worshipped") femmes, where all they praised was high femme aesthetic choices—the five-inch heels, the perfect winged eyeliner. Never pain. Never imperfection. Never mess. But what about when you're a femme and you're too depressed and fucked up to perfect that eyeliner wing? What about when you're femme and suicidal and you've been in the same sleep pants that smell bad for weeks?

I have never seen a masculine person write an ode to how much they love their femme partner or friend when s/he is in sweatpants that smell bad. I have rarely seen a hymn to femmes who are fucked up and failing, not available, driving everyone nuts, including ourselves. I thought about all the femmes I know, including myself, whose hands shake too much to do eyeliner. Are we loved by our communities when we're unable to accomplish the high femme aesthetics that are all many people know how to name as femme? Are we loved when we are "ugly"? So much of the time, my experiences in queer community show that we are not invisible; we are often hyper-visible, but our femme identities and lives are often erased, disrespected, and profoundly misunderstood. Crazy femme times are some of those times when our lived experiences of scarred femmeness are not our communities' default of the "strong femmes" they love to "worship" but the sad femmes they don't always know how to love.

Femme armor can also be a prison. So many of us survive on this thin edge of barbwire life by looking like we have it all together. Our femme armor is a way we protect ourselves. The perfect lip, hair on point, brows too, outfits curated as works of art, charms, and amulets. All of this, magic to keep the assholes away. If your nails are done, you can feel like something is under control, even if everything is falling apart. Your lip insists on respect. Your makeup makes sure you're not clocked as trans. You presentation is labor that makes you the money you need.

Yet my friend Naima Lowe says, "Armor can also be a prison." If only armor insists and wins our rights to be respected in love, when crazy comes, we might not know that we are also loved in sweat and tears and mess and undone. One of the biggest pieces of love I have seen are the places where femmes—mostly poor and working class and disabled—give each other this love and permission to be messy. It's thin on the ground everyplace else.

Femmes who are in community leadership are targets for huge amounts of rage and abuse. Success is not a protection from suicide. Femmes get suicidal when everything "looks great"—I got suicidal when I had just won a Lambda. That can be both because madness strikes for many reasons at many times (including chronically) and because succeeding makes one vulnerable to attack and rage as much as praise. I've seen femmes who do, well, just about anything—organize a show or start a counseling practice or throw a workshop or a conference or a political action—be subject to both an incredible amount of rage and abuse hurled at them if they make a mistake or if anything is not 100 percent pleasing to 100% of the people 100% of the time, *and* a huge expectation that they be 1,000% available to listen, soothe, apologize, and drop everything to talk that rage out. People seem, for some wild reason (you know, sexism), to feel they have more of a license to lash out in rage at femmes when their steak is not cooked perfectly.

This well-known and little-discussed fact has a huge impact on femme mental health. Many femmes I know are survivors of abuse—nerds and weirdos who suffered from homophobia, growing up in ways we might not even have had words for, because the real dykes were masculine, right? We are also femmes of color, poor and working-class femmes, disabled femmes, sex-working femmes. We start community projects not necessarily to get fame and fortune but to try to save lives or fulfill a crucial need. Often, we make ourselves vulnerable as part of that work. We have been raised to stay humble and accessible, or value that as a principle of accountable community leadership. And when we do something, the assumption is often *Who does ze think ze is?* Our humility, accessibility, and openness make us vulnerable to attack. So often, we have not been taught that it's okay to have boundaries, say no, that we can be accountable without being 1,000% perfect all the time, that we can be leaders who get to make mistakes. Worse, our work isn't seen as real anyway.

I have almost never heard a femme leader admit or speak openly about the impact these attacks have had on their spirit. Yet a hell of a lot of femmes have spoken to me privately of the depression, anxiety, and PTSD that have come from being femmes in visible leadership. If the only place we and our gender are loved is on a pedestal, and one mistake throws us off the pedestal into a pit of hell ... well, that's not a recipe for anything like love, or liberation.

So many people say, "I had no idea" when someone dies. I think we have to ask ourselves, "Why didn't we"? What is okay to talk about in these places we call queer community? What isn't? It's not enough to say, "Just call." I think that we could use suicidal deaths in our communities to interrogate the shit out of how saneism and ableism are diffused throughout queer community.

In so many hip queer communities that are not explicitly disabled, it's not okay to not be okay. We pay lip service, but how many times do you ask someone how they're doing at a party and hear anything besides how great things are going, or feel like you can be honest about how things are really going for you?

I was actively suicidal for my last several years living in the Bay Area. Part of what contributed to my suicidality was the headfuck of living in a place so beautiful, held up to be a certain kind of queer of color utopia but where there was a lot of lip service paid to community, mutual aid, and care. The Bay was filled with beautiful people, multiple queer dance parties every night, an emphasis on a youthful party culture of bacchanalia and pleasure. But what happened when you were too sick or sad to make it to the dance party? Too often, you disappeared from mattering to that public community of queerness.

And what happens when this is what you know of how queer community exists? When you feel too crazy to make it to the pretty dance party, you may feel like there is no place for you at all. When you don't know—because it is systematically invisibilized—that there is queer crip community happening in beds, living rooms, coffee shops, on Skype, and it counts just as much. I've had my life saved by prioritizing queer disabled people of color friendship. But I know that most non-disabled QTBIPOC community has no idea that disabled queer of color communities exist.

FEMME EMOTIONAL SAFETY STRATEGIES FOR SURVIVAL AND BEYOND

In fall 2016, after the spate of femme suicides, me, Maryse Mitchell-Brody, Naima Lowe, Kai Cheng Thom, and Elena Rose, decided to try to do something about it.

The Femme Emotional Safety Strategies for Survival and Beyond webinars (or femminars) were online spaces by and for queer femmes to discuss suicidality in our lives and the lives of others.[54] We collaborated with the Icarus Project, a radical mental health network founded by two white non-femme people, whose departure a few years previous had kicked off a process to change Icarus from a white, punk, often racist and sexist community group to one that centered racial and gender justice. Icarus's new part-time staff was a mix of femmes of color: one straight, immigrant single mom living in the South and one working-class queer white woman. We got a microgrant to pay facilitators and started letting folks know about the program. In the first week, 400 people signed up, and many people expressed desperate feelings of gratitude that, as one femme put it, "There was

54   For archived and transcribed videos of the femminars, see the Icarus Project, https://vimeo.com/theicarusproject.

an organized, intentional response" to the femme deaths. I agreed, and I also raged—why had it taken so long?

We worked for many more than the hours we had funding to pay people for teaching the curriculum for the general Black-and-brown-femme-only and trans-women/trans-feminine-only femminars. The femminars were a rare space for femmes to come together to talk suicide, "mental health," crisis and death. Almost everyone who signed up said they were doing it because they wanted to know how to support someone else. There were nods of recognition, tears, and raised fists when we talked about some of what we saw happening for femmes who were suicidal. One femme added that they had seen many occasions of femmes with masculine partners and friends who stuck by the masculine person through crisis after crisis, only to have that person say, "Sorry, I can't do this" and then leave when the femme had a crisis of their own. When we asked folks what they did to stay alive, the answers were a rainbow femme quilt of femme emotional intelligence. Meds Netflix therapy prayer herbs change breakups fresh nails praying to the ancestors breaking bottles finding a friend you can be crazy with shutting down social media reaching out on social media groups that felt safe crying baths all the crystals shit talk. All little things that weren't so little. It struck me, watching them, how easily they might be called "nothing" by the outside world. Minimized, like femmes are.

And when Maryse ended one femminar by saying, "It is totally okay to do emotional labor for yourself first," I let out a breath I didn't know I'd been holding.

A few weeks before the femminars launched, and three days after Trump was elected president, I traveled to my hometown of Toronto. There I met with Carly Boyce, a white, genderqueer femme who had been organizing workshops "about how to be there for your friends who are freaks and weirdos who sometimes want to die." I was curious about their process and experiences and wanted to share what we were thinking and doing with ours. We talked about our beliefs about suicide. I shared mine, one that has kept me alive since I was a teenager, that I gleaned from radical abuse survivors and Indigenous feminist organizers and friends: the idea that suicide was a weapon of the abuser and the colonizer, a bomb they plant in our bodies to try to kill us, and that it was political for me to fight to survive and live.

Carly listened and shared an alternate view: to them, the idea of preventing suicide at all costs risked becoming like pro-lifers who fight to save every fetal "life" but do nothing to support children and parents once children are born. If we were going to insist on fighting to keep our people here, Carly said, we also had to work on shifting conditions to allow people to be able to stay. Otherwise, insisting that "everyone needs to promise to live!" without actually changing the conditions that make people want to die is an ableist setup that hangs suicidal folks out to dry. The same way that transformative justice argues that we must change the conditions that caused people to harm in order to heal the harm that happened and prevent it from happening again, Carly pushed for addressing the root causes of suicidality—something more of a long-term project than the immediate crisis response most folks tend to know how to react with when someone is suicidal.

GRIEF CAN BE THE GARDEN: A FEMME SUICIDE ALTAR

Taueret's photo on the card from her memorial—one of her many iconic poses, full lips parted, direct stance and stare, nameplate necklace—stares at me every day from my altar to where I write on my cripbed. Her glance is a challenge. And a dare. Her image sits next to an 8.5″-by-11″ print of roses growing in the courtyard of a housing project with the words GRIEF CAN BE THE GARDEN floating above. I bought the print at a QTBIPOC comic and zine fair in Seattle after a 2016 filled to the brim with annealing grief.

The two images speak to each other, and to me. If grief can be the garden. If femme suicide and death can be loss, and can also be a sign pointing to what needs to change. I want to grow femme communities where we do not have to be perfect to thrive. Where there are a million ways of being femme, and femme is less about being perfect and never about being pedestalized. Where femme labor and intelligence are recognized and rewarded instead of mocked, punished, and ignored. Where people realize that femme does not automatically and unconsensually equal Mommy. Where we rebuild how femme is seen, understood, cherished. Where we use all our femme suicide science to figure out how to live, and we share it with all genders of people to support each other figuring out how to live and resist well. Where the dance party is at home and messy and in sweatpants. Where I don't have to be cool to be worth fighting for or legible or seen.

I've never yet seen a masculine person write that love letter to messy, suicidal, perfect femmes, but here is mine:

> *Femmes, I love you when your hands shake too much from meds or stress or disability to put on eyeliner, let alone put it on perfectly. I love you when you don't wear eyeliner. I love you when you are deeply sad, raging, in despair, not "pretty," in the same sweats for three days or a month, when you smell like sweat and fear and the deep sad. I love you when you cough up phlegm. I love you when you scream and rage and ache. I love you when you don't wear those five-inch heels because your feet hurt or it's a sexier choice as a disabled femme to wear kicks (like the gold glitter ones I am wearing right now). And I want a community where we can be messy, in pain, hurting, imperfect, and we really know that our genders are still seen and cherished.*

Two or three things I know about femme suicide, and they are:

I believe in fighting for femmes to stay alive. I believe fighting for us to live is a revolutionary act.

I believe that when we shift conditions of ableism, femmephobia, sexism, classism, transmisogyny, fatphobia, and whorephobia, everyone gets more free and safe and able to stay.

I believe in femmes first. I believe in crazy femmes first.

I want us to live. I mean to survive, and I can't do it alone.

My grief about femme suicide is the garden where our future grows.

PART
IV

FOR BADASS DISABILITY JUSTICE, WORKING-CLASS AND POOR-LED MODELS OF SUSTAINABLE HUSTLING FOR LIBERATION

B. Loewe's piece "An End to Self Care" made me really angry and really scared when it came out in 2012.[55] For folks who need a reminder or missed it the first time, "An End to Self Care" is an article where white, nonbinary, able-bodied labor organizer B. Loewe argues against any focus on care and healing in radical movements, seeing it as a form of weakness in organizing. The first thing that gave me the feelings? B.'s anecdote about Don Andres, a working-class brown man who didn't need "self-care" because going to a meeting after a day labor workday that began at six a.m. was his self-care.

Here's the thing: middle- or upper-class organizers from the 1800s to now just loooooooove painting majestic, romanticized, simplistic pictures of poor and working class people. Hint: we're not all one thing. We are amazing, diverse, complicated in our poverty and working-class scholarship. My life as the kid of a working-class Irish/Roma rust belt mom who grew up in recession Massachusetts in the 1980s and who won a bunch of scholarships is real different from my friend who grew up the daughter of a poverty-class, sex-working, white mama in the '80s. And that's the great thing—as broke folks, we get to have conversations with each other about all the different things being

---

55   B. Lowe, "An End to Self Care" *Organizing Upgrade*, October 15, 2012, http://archive. organizingupgrade.com/index.php/component/k2/item/729-end-to-self-care, accessed June 5, 2018.

poor or working class has meant to us, looked like to us, taught us, gifted us with, and our genius, which could give birth to entirely new galaxies of movements and forms of organizing. (Sarcasm definitely in there, and definitely may only be picked up on by other folks who were raised poor or working class.) Sometimes, anyway. There are so many things that make it difficult for us to find each other.

One thing I know for sure we aren't? Cardboard cutout workers who work selflessly for the movement seventeen or eighteen hours a day, handing out leaflets. In middle- and upper-middle-class writing about broke folks, we're always either noble, selfless, salt-of-the-earth worker warriors with nary a sensitive need to be found or lumpen, loud, rude-ass, stupid criminals and welfare class. We don't get to speak for ourselves—especially about how brutalizing classist stereotypes about our lives like these are, *and* how these stereotypes affect the health of our poor and working-class minds, bodies, and spirits. Or about the ways we find to care for ourselves every day, how we struggle against how "self-care" has been defined as a luxury for white and middle/upper-class people. Salt of This Earth would look reaaaaal different if it was written by and for street-involved, poverty-class, femme of color sex workers.

So in the meantime, while we're trying to find each other to have those conversations? Maybe don't write about working-class/poor folks as if you know what our experiences are from the inside—especially when it's something as deeply complex as issues of work, hustle, need, softness, our tough and vulnerable bodies. 'Cause that brown farmworking man who got up at six a.m.? Maybe he did want some sleep. Some community acupuncture. A limpia. Some love. Maybe he's got it. Maybe he's not talking about that stuff to you because it's real personal.

Oh, working-class and poor folks hustle our asses off, sure we do. I've had multiple jobs and hustles for as long as I can remember. I always have fifteen things on the go. Guess what else I have? A chronic illness and disability that don't allow me to get out on the picket line eighteen hours a day. Guess what else I have? Badass resilience strategies of loud-ass working-class, femme of color laughter and shit-talking; organizing methods with other disabled and/or chronically ill folks who find ways to do amazing organizing that centers what our bodies can actually do; trading massages as we sit in court praying for a youth who's been locked up on bullshit charges, doing grounding and praying to our ancestors outside court, a spiritual practice that is banging; doing yoga every morning in my house, for free, that allows me to manage my pain, fatigue, and cognitive challenges and helps me do my work from a grounded place of love that centers my crip body. I could add: good food that is cooked by me and my (queer, brown, disabled) housemates, herbs that are cheap brewing in a mason jar on my stove, and a sense of what I can do well and how much time it actually takes to do it. Disabled imperfect collective care models that are works in progress but still show up, with folks who help each other with personal care, rides to the grocery store, hanging out to combat total isolation. Shared rides and money. Shared resources. These are working-class/poor, POC, disabled, and femme strategies for self and collective care. Because it's not either/or.

There's something deep I want to tease out here—about working-class and poor folks and work. Some of us, we work so hard. We work so much. We don't sleep. We don't stop. We have our own somatics, a way of being in our bodies, of toughness and sucking it up and making it happen. We do it because we have to, because we love it, because it's a way of saying fuck you to everyone who's ever said we're lazy and it's our fault we don't have money. And this can be a gift. And it can also kill us. *And* there's so much in here about care and sensitivity and being able to breathe being coded as luxuries for the wealthy. *And* what about folks who are on SSI, unemployed, too sick to work?

What about the complex interplay between labor and pain and our bodies and how poor and working-class bodies are supposedly too tough to feel anything? Yet we do. Deeply. And in much talk about sustainability, there's not enough talk about how we, as broke/disabled folks, do it—what sustainability means to us.

Yes, self-care—like non-Western, non-biomedical models of healing—has been co-opted by people who want to make money off it. And typical burnout movement organizations that are, maybe, starting to try a little bit to not run their workers into the ground 'til they get sick, sometimes they do the same work at the same breakneck crisis pace they've done it, and then take them away for a four-day yoga retreat. But that's not actually using a model of sustainability that comes from disability justice! It's doing the same kind of organizing nonprofit-industrial complex movements have insisted on for years—which pushes out parents, broke folks, and disabled folks, to name just a few, but tacks on a little self-care on the side.

Getting rid of yoga is not the solution. Listening to broke-ass, disabled, and femme communities about how we actually create ways of organizing where we're not just grinding ourselves into the dust *and* we're not going on some $4,000 spa vacation once a year might be.

"We can't knit our way to revolution," Loewe says. Oh yeah? Wow, what a femmephobic and classist statement. Many, many people have organized politically through cultural work—which includes knitting and quilting bees—for a very long time. I think it's a problem how Lowe dismisses this femme-identified form of cultural creation (and just managing your anxiety and making a sweater for your kid during a meeting). I think conversation and mutual support is a particular form of organizing that is often a femme organizing skill (not that other genders can't also do this) that isn't valued or witnessed enough in organizing because of sexism and femmephobia and transmisogyny. I think that knitting through meetings, and creating an organizational culture where that's seen as badass, is something that many of my badass working-class femme of color and white femme organizers do. But Loewe has a point I agree with—maybe the one they hoped would be picked up the most. It's the point that collective care should be lifted up, that self-care shouldn't just be this individualized bourgie thing. But I wish Lowe'd had any kind of disability justice model in their article at all. I wish they hadn't reified this idea of good movement work as going back to an eighty-hour-a-week hustle. I wish they hadn't gone right into "self-care is just for the privileged, look at this noble worker on the corner, he doesn't need yoga" stance.

Sure, movements can be healing. But are they? Many, many broke folks, parents, and/or disabled folks who have been forced out of movements would say no. What disability justice and healing justice talks about—and asks—is: Are they really? Or are they set up in burnout models that destroy folks' physical and spiritual health? And I think that a big part of what movements I'm part of do to make movements that aren't shitty is centering disabled, working-class and poor, parenting, and femme of color genius. Burnout isn't just about not having a deep enough analysis. It's about movements that are deeply ableist and inaccessible.

Like many disabled and chronically ill folks, Loewe's article terrified me. As able-bodied organizer after organizer posted it on Facebook with glowing praise, all I could think of was the ripple effect of reinforcing ableism—already vastly present, like air, in movements and completely ignored (as a crip, you get used to the blank look nondisabled activists give you when you try to talk about ableism, access, that disabled people aren't just tragic or heroic, etc.)—and how people using this article to shit-talk "self-care" was going to make shit so much worse for folks with disabilities and chronic illnesses, parents, and caretakers trying to be activists. Including folks who have chronic health and disability, but who are deeply in the closet about it because they're terrified of losing their jobs or activist cred or self-worth if they come out as disabled. This is just one example of how I want non-disabled activists to be accountable—for real—about making fighting ableism central in everything we do, and to pay attention to how invisibilized anti-ableism struggles are in a lot of mainstream social justice work.

I'm used to people saying to me, "Wow, your self-care is so good!" I always look at them blankly. I never think of what I do—cooking good food for myself on my budget that supports my body and my chronic illness, going to working-class acupuncture twice a month, stretching, drinking a lot of herbs, making sure I get sleep—as "self-care." I think of it as the stuff I do to love myself in a fucked-up world, to help me have more days with less pain, and to help me give my body love when I'm having days with a lot of pain and fatigue.

Let's tease it out further—when my friends who use power wheelchairs need a personal care attendant many times a day to pee and transfer from bed to chair, is that "self-care"? It's not commonly thought of that way—but it's part of the whole continuum of *bodily need* that gets trashed as a pain in the ass by an ableist world. Loewe writes, "I have literally gone from being in debilitating pain and only being able to accomplish three hours of work each day to working 18 hour shifts the same week in a completely different context. The difference was not the conditions of my work. It was my connection to my purpose." I'm glad that works for them. But, as a friend of mine remarked, "Okay, that method does not work for some of us. Some of us are in debilitating pain no matter what." And to say that we can just be "more deeply committed to the struggle" and leave our disabilities behind is an incredibly dangerous, ableist stance to take—that also just plain ignores the reality that *some people are just disabled and can't think or organize our way to able-bodiedness.*

But we can do things differently, as organizers. We do it all the time. For example, that moment I mentioned before—us massaging each other in court while witnessing and supporting a youth who'd been locked up under gang injunction and anti-terrorism laws? That really happened, to a student. We came together as a community to raise money for her lawyer, spread the word, support her family, show up in court, and much more.

Now, we could've done this in a typical movement burnout way—speed, panic, conference calls, panic, no food or breath or sleep. But instead, we prayed to our ancestors at the rally before her first day in court. We cooked for each other. Knowing that many people at the rally had either been locked up or had loved ones who are, and being inside the courthouse could be really hard, a community member led us all in a somatic grounding so we could feel our bodies' power before we went into the courthouse. We shared food and rides and supported each other. There was always a feeling that if people couldn't make it because of work or parenting or disability/illness, other folks would move up.

This is the kind of movement I want to be part of. I want movements to embody a disabled, working-class, brown sustainability that celebrates femme organizer genius. We deserve nothing less. And we—disabled, working-class femmes of color—have been creating these kinds of movements for a long time. Listen up. (Or read the captioning.)

PROTECT YOUR HEART

FEMME LEADERSHIP AND HYPER-ACCOUNTABILITY

The summer and fall of 2015, I lived in Brooklyn. I had moved there pretty rapidly from Toronto when I got together with my partner, who was born, raised, and living in Queens. I had had a lot of long-distance relationships at that point in my life, and I didn't want any more. If we were going to be any kind of distance, we were going to be a cross-borough, 7 to the G train kinda distance relationship.

That summer and fall, there was a graffiti stencil I noticed everywhere—down my block and in the Lower East Side. *Protect Your Heart*, it said. It reminded me of a line of Black, queer, HIV-positive poet Essex Hemphill's: "protect your magic."

I felt like it was showing up then for a reason. Those words appeared at a time when I was healing from and getting perspective about a lot of shit that had gone down in my thirties—about some people who I had worked with for a long time who had acted in ways I was starting to recognize as emotionally abusive. Realizing this also made me look at how hyper-accountability in my life as a disabled femme of color survivor had been a superpower and a survival skill—and also something that had almost killed me.

A common idea in social justice culture is that if someone calls you out on being oppressive, you need to shut up, listen, put aside your automatic defensive reaction, and accept what they're saying, learn from it, and thank them. This is a useful ground rule, and it works for a lot of situations. We've all seen White Nonsense people clutch their pearls and deny they have privilege. Or cis people or abled people or non–sex workers or whatever. And also, people with all kinds of oppressions fuck up too and need to get told we're fucking up.

But there's also a line between setting aside defensiveness and being open to hearing how you've fucked up or hurt someone without knee-jerking to "You're wrong! I'm perfect! Fuck you!" and letting someone walk all over you and emotionally abuse and gaslight you.

And, sometimes, when you're some combination of survivor, femme, and a mix of oppressions, you can have been raised to automatically be accountable for every single thing. It rained? I'm sorry. You're stressed? It's my fault. Let me fix it. You didn't like the show? You're right, I'm totally fucked up.

And you can end up in a place where people are "coming for you" in ways that cross the line from justifiably angry to abusive and can have a lot of consequences. Consequences that have landed many femme of color leaders I know with PTSD, anxiety, trauma, suicidality, and more. Have set us up to be abused or landed us in situations of abuse we didn't know how to call abuse. Have made us move away from leadership or activism because it hurt too much and one day our hearts just gave up.

Some fast facts about me: I am a supersurvivor. For some of you, that phrase will be enough, but in case it's not, let me spell it out: I've had horrible things done to my body and mind, sexually and emotionally, as a very young child and a preteen, a teenager and an adult. I am an empath. I am neurodivergent, and I see things in pictures and feelings long before the words come. I can read pain face and trauma face on other people from a million feet away. I supported my mom who was a survivor and also someone who caused harm and a crip (even though she would never call herself that) through her suicidality when I was a kid, her only child, and the only person she trusted.

Because of that, I am very fast—in comprehension, in knowing what you're feeling, in knowing something is wrong. I have superpowers: I know what you're feeling before you feel it. I am the best smoke detector, fire alarm, CO detector money can't buy. I am a first responder. I run towards the burning building, and I rush to give the remedy.

I've been praised for it all my life, this thing now being called femme emotional labor that is also crip, crazy, and survivor. And I have internalized that it is my job and my worth, the thing I am skilled at doing, the thing that was my value when I was not seen as pretty or worthy of protection.

Also, I think if I or you say what needs to be said just the right way, the world will be saved and the revolution will come and I won't die. Also, I have complex PTSD, DID, and a bunch of other stuff, so, as my friend who also has all of these things says, "I'm easy to fuck with." If you tell me I did something, I will be like, "Wait, what happened? Did I say that?" I also have a lot of panic from being neurodivergent and not understanding it for years, of, *Fuck, did the words fuck up again because they got lost in meaning-to-spoken-language translation again? I'm a freak and I'm in trouble now and people are mad!* So I try real hard to get it all right. And I get really, really stressed out in that somatic FIGHT FLIGHT FREEZE APPEASE TO THE DEATH limbic brain way when I think I maybe have not gotten it right.

Finally, I am a survivor who has not had people listen to or believe me about my experiences, at some really crucial times that resulted in me almost dying. So, what that's led me towards is a place where I don't ever want anyone who's been harmed to not have me, or anyone, believe that they've been harmed. Ever.

Your story might be different. But my guess is a good chunk of folks reading this have your own version, or know what I'm talking about anyway. The world of radicals and queers is filled with people who survived by doing all of the above, and then brought it to social justice movements. Maybe you were trained for different reasons to know and care about other people's needs and wants before you ever felt your own. Maybe you've been on the other side of the coin.

So there has been this dynamic I've witnessed and participated in:

Survivor, QTBIPOC, often femme in some way, often disabled or poor/working-class, empath, weirdo genius decides to try and Do a Thing—to Do What Needs to Be Done, and to also be useful, and maybe because they are also gifted at it, and like it, and want to write/organize/sing/heal/whatever. Someone who also maybe does this work coming from a history of not being valued. Who thinks, maybe if I am useful, I won't be thrown away.

And then:

Things get created. Shows, spaces, resources, etc. It's gorgeous. The organizer gets some attention for it. There are many emails asking questions, for support, for things, giving feedback, asking for more.

And after that:

The thing that is created, it's great but not perfect. Some criticisms come in and are real. But also, said femme empathic person is on the receiving end of a butt-ton of hate, blog posts that go on for six pages about how fucked up the thing is, in detail. There are online flame wars and long emails that make a lot of assumptions and have few ground rules.

And finally:

The person attacking (and sometimes the femme being attacked too—basically, everyone involved) believes that to be "accountable," the femme in question is not allowed to have any boundaries or filters. They are not allowed to take a minute to think about it. The only allowable response is to automatically apologize and agree.

When I write and think about femme suicidality, one thing I think about is this kind of intense, compound pressure we are under. I have had many private conversations with femmes doing cultural, healing, or political organizing work who've shared that their depression, anxiety, and suicidality skyrocketed as they did work and became seen as visible "leaders." This is ironic, because we're taught in radical community that doing the work and getting good at it is part of what will heal us. But the work they did, a lot of it healed them and was amazing. But also, it meant that some people became enraged at them—when they disagreed with them, when the emailed reply didn't come fast enough, or when someone made a mistake. The people who were pissed—sometimes people of all genders, sometimes other femmes—came at them in really intense ways, often publicly, telling them how fucked up they were. Sometimes, this happened when there was a legit fuckup and people were justifiably angry; sometimes, the confrontation came from a place that was also about rage and jealousy and bullying.

(And now I must pause for a moment and say: It's immensely complex to try to talk about online attack and the "callout culture" wars, and it makes me tired even thinking about trying to talk about it. To some folks, any voiced anger online plays into "disposability culture"; to some, any request that they take it down a notch is censorship. However, here is my brief attempt at Leah Lakshmi's Universal Theorem of Online Calling Out: I think that oppressed people have a right to tell the person doing the oppressing to get their foot off their necks. I think that anger is valid, and that many people, particularly Black, Indigenous, people of color, fat, working-class, and disabled people, get told we need to say it nicer when we're mad at things that aren't right, and that kind of tone policing is wrong. I also think there are times when people are capable of doing emotionally abusive, completely out-of-pocket shit online that is destructive and crazy-making in the name of confrontation. I think that working things out is often great; I also think that sometimes people have a right to set boundaries, including cutting people the fuck off. I think trauma, abuse, and oppression have made it so we often have zero experience of anything other than betrayal, so the safest way we know how to survive is to rip someone's face off or run. I think there is no hard-and-fast rule—one person's clusterfuck is another person's righteous call for justice. All I can do is rely on my own internal sense of what feels right and ask friends for reality checks. A lot of things can be true at the same time. You're welcome.)

I have not heard of this same experience, at the same rate, occurring to masculine leaders. I have not witnessed there being the same expectation that masculine leaders in queer social justice communities must be 1,000% emotionally accessible all the time, write back to every Facebook message immediately and perfectly, listen, support, and apologize. What seems real is that people have both more entitled expectations of femmes' time and ears, and of femmes being perfect. Expectations run high that you are either a magic mommy who fixes everything perfectly and infallibly and never says no, or you are a shit failure bitch who deserves every bit of rage thrown at you. There is also a sense that it is okay and easy to be violent and/or raging towards the femme in question—both rooted in sexism and femmephobia. After all, what is Mommy for but to be screamed at? What is femininity under the WSCCAP but to be perfect or to be abused?

Some of the people who have come for me have gotten the angriest when I've been too tired or sick or just otherwise occupied to drop everything to engage. Have told me to stop "making excuses." But when someone is legit sick, cripped out, exhausted, or nuts, isn't it actually responsible to own those things, attend to them, and then make a different space to come together to deal with whatever happened? Isn't it ableist to tell someone to just stop being disabled already? Aren't there ways we can create where we can be sick and tired and nuts and accountable in an accessible way?

When people ask me why I moved away from Oakland after living there for most of my thirties, I usually stick to what's easiest to tell: that I got priced out of living there because of Google and other tech companies driving up rent, and I had been away from home for a long time and needed to go back.

All of those things are true. The reason that is harder to talk about is that I lived with pretty deep depression the last four years in Oakland. Depression that could, and did, flare into suicidality and chronic anxiety and panic. There were a number of reasons for my mental health going down the toilet, but two big ones were that I was on the receiving end of some relationships that had become emotionally abusive, that I didn't even know how to name as such, and that I was doing an incredible amount of emotional labor and I didn't know that I was allowed to have any limits around it. I didn't know how to also say that it felt not only like some of the folks I'd been the closest with in the Bay didn't love, know, or respect me but also like they actively wanted me to go down. I had thought I had come to the QTBIPOC promised land, and it hurt here too. I was often afraid to leave the house, to go to shows or events. Every time I looked at my email or Facebook and saw a message, my first thought was whether someone was angry at me. Every single thing was urgent. Every single thing was an emergency, at the same rate.

After I moved, back to Toronto in the middle of a long quiet winter, some things became clearer. For one, a huge percentage of the unpaid femme emotional labor I was doing fell away. From 2010 to 2014, I had been living in collective houses of six to ten people, which was often an unpaid twenty-hour-a-week job. Talking to everyone while trying to get dressed, doing everyone's dishes so I had some to cook with, dealing with slumlord conditions—roofs caving in, pipes exploding, break-ins, racist white men doing racist white performance art at house open mics—all of it took hours of spoons. I was also a member of at least two collectives and did hours and hours of unpaid labor in them: creating websites, organizing meetings, organizing events, answering emails, fundraising. I worked multiple jobs for money, most of which involved some kind of intensive trauma-infused care work—from teaching med students how to do sexual health exams in a consent-based and trauma-aware model to co-running a QTBIPOC performance collective to teaching and talking about rape, transformative justice, and intimate partner violence. I was part of friend and online disability communities where I did an enormous amount of caretaking and support work. I did huge unpaid roles running some things at some annual conferences and gathering spaces. Plus, oh yes, I had a small counseling practice. And on top of it all came the hyper-accountability I speak of—the place of, with all of these things, feeling like I had to be constantly available and accessible to deal with critique, communication, feedback, etc.

Everyone I knew was doing the exact same rate of work, to survive being low income, queer, Black or brown, and sick and disabled in a skyrocketing gentrification economy. And, hey, it was all fun and for the revolution and I was lucky to be able to do it instead of being normal, right? And it was literally keeping me alive, right? I was cash poor—something I rarely talked about, because I was clear about my privileges, like light skin and citizenship and access to higher education, scholarship or not. But I was also living on less than $1,200 a month with no stable income but five to six part-time accessible-ish gigs. I wholeheartedly believed that what I had going for me, especially in all my sick/bed time, was being hyper-available—being spooned out on Facebook but offering care both to support my community and to have the hope of receiving care and support back when I needed it. There were also so many working-class values—that showing up is just what you do, for example—in this pattern. Aside from a few Resource Generation kids or trust fund kids (whom I mostly didn't hang out with, because rich people get on my nerves), I didn't know anyone who even approached a middle-class standard of living. We all were hustling, and we all had an ethic of sharing the hustle. The free box and the crowdfund would save you. There were also definitely some elements of being the child of a mother who was working class and suicidal, who raised me to be her counselor and confidante and best friend, the keeper of secrets, the empathic, smart, autistic kid who knew her feelings before she did.

So I had no idea how to see all of this labor as work, or to see that perhaps I might need some days off or some—what do you call them?—limits. I had no idea any of this was stressful. I had no idea any of this was "work." I sort of understood why I was so anxious and exhausted all the time but not really. It was what everyone I knew was doing, and I just thought of it as the right thing to do. I would, however, frequently lie in my bed on my heating pad in mid-flare, watching Netflix half-heartedly, truly feeling that if I dropped dead very few people would notice until I didn't show up for a meeting.

I had no idea of any of this—that all of this labor really was work, that I was tired from working hard, not from being lazy; that I might need some quiet and space; that being hyper-accessible was killing me—until I moved back to Toronto, and ninety percent of that work dropped away. Those collectives were thousands of miles away, and I was living with mostly just one other person for one fragile second. And I felt ... well, peaceful.

All of a sudden, I had a lot more time. And choices. And quiet. And my mental health? It got better. A lot better. I was loved, even when I wasn't working. I had time to cry. I had time to think. I was pretty much around people I liked, who liked me. And I was like, wow. All of that work. That was work. All of that abuse. That was abuse.

For a while I didn't have the words, to say how toxic and hard it was to live in a city where community was talked about constantly, but in actuality there was a lot of rage and shallowness, where if you weren't pretty, popular, and full of energy, people could not give much of a shit about you. It hurt worse because I had drunk the Bay Area Kool-Aid—that this was a place of love, feelings, and healing. I had come there to make it, to be a performer and producer, and I had. But I also felt attacked in what I had staked my life on. And I want to talk about that—about what happens when you merge identity and work inside a politicized community.

I was raised pretty feral, in a family with a lot of abuse and a lot of neurodivergence that led to a lot of isolation. There was a lot we weren't supposed to speak about outside the home, there were a lot of secrets, and there was a lot of fear of The World. From when I was a kid, I decided I wanted the world, and I wanted to grow up to have a big family and a big house. This was especially important to me because I knew that I was probably going to have to run really hard from my parents, and I was going to lose my biological family.

As a young adult, I survived some pretty intense things—almost getting killed by an abusive partner, leaving the country, having my parents threaten to get me institutionalized when I told them about the childhood sexual abuse I was remembering, having a partner who was also my immigration sponsor threaten to kill me and stalk me for years, and being very sick with a serious chronic illness.

During those years when I was very sick, very crazy, very poor, and very in a physically abusive relationship, I almost died from the isolation. I did not have social capital. I was poor, not pretty, could not stop talking about the abuse I was experiencing and was just starting to have survived, and was sick with a chronic illness during a period of little to no disability community or respect for disability within social justice communities. Everybody was young and able-bodied and normalesque.

Part of the way I rebuilt my place in my city, as I got slightly less sick, as I was able to work legally, was by being helpful. I did not believe that I was valued in and of myself, for myself. I was not pretty or normal or unscarred. But I started doing a lot of social justice service work. I started queer youth writing circles, wrote poetry, organized things. I believed in community, forever. I believed in always working things out with friend family. I worked very hard to have no conflict with anyone and to immediately smooth over any conflict that happened. I worked very hard and was very generous. I believed that if I proved myself to be indispensable, to be useful, I would not be thrown away, I would have a place, I would be useful and thus loved, or something like loved, because my inside parts were not lovable but my usefulness was.

I built a writing career, partly out of these underpinnings. I became a community-based writer, who was writing for my community, and also for myself. I embraced the ideas of community-based poet as people's newspaper, journalist, tool-crafter—as someone who worked and wrote for the people, so the people were my boss. I didn't have a family, so I was committed, in a really intense, my life depends on it, orphan freak way, to being loved by "community." For my writing to be a career. For me to feel of any value or use.

That's very common. It's also dangerous.

No one told me I could have a filter. No one told me that it was impossible to be liked by everyone. No one told me that it was okay to have a private life, or to say no to some requests for information. No one told me I could write for the community but also write from my own sense of what I wanted and needed to write, and that I could tell the community to fuck off sometimes. No one told me I didn't have to take every critique or comment at 100 percent face value. No one warned me that some folks would just lash out because of jealousy or being triggered or rage. No one told me I wasn't a bad person if I couldn't answer every single email or message telling me I was fucked up. No one told me that if a stranger, or a semi stranger, attacked me, I could protect myself, I didn't have to answer, I could have a limit, I didn't have to offer them my throat. No one told me I could make art and do work but also be loved and valued on my own terms, not just for being useful, for doing labor, for being in leadership.

This is my story, but it's so many other people's stories.

No one told me. But I tell myself now. And I tell other femme, working-class, disabled leaders today: protect your heart.

It is okay if you build in boundaries.

It is okay if you are imperfect.

It is okay and good to build relationships where you are loved not just for your labor.

It is okay to say no to being everyone's mommy.

It is okay to not reply to everyone's email instantaneously.

It is okay to build relationships with the expectation that you both will make mistakes and you get to make amends and repair.

If someone comes shooting, you can give yourself some cover, not hand them your heart.

You are a renewable and also limited resource.

You deserve to be held.

NOT OVER IT, NOT FIXED, AND LIVING A LIFE WORTH LIVING

TOWARDS AN ANTI-ABLEIST VISION OF SURVIVORHOOD

To all survivors today: your time is precious, your energy is precious, you are precious. Your love is precious, your relationships are precious. And I don't mean precious like cute. I mean precious like invaluable like massive like power like transcendent.
—Hannah Harris-Sutro

Healing is dangerous work. Healing is about going into the struggle. When trauma happens, we go away from that space in our body where it happened—and when we go into it, it hurts so much as it wakes back up. I'm interested in creating the place where the body can remember itself, even though it hurts to do it. Where feeling better is part of it, but it's not the goal. Struggling better is the goal.
—Susan Raffo

UNFIXED, EVADING CAPTURE

Recently, I was auditioning a new therapist who, during the intake interview, asked me in all sincerity, "So, do you think the therapy you got in your twenties resolved your childhood sexual abuse?"

I stared at her with my mouth open for a solid thirty seconds.

I'd had such high hopes for that therapist. She was a woman of color with a Cesar Chavez quote on her website; she worked at the local healing justice center. She said she was "trauma-informed" and listed working with survivors as one of her areas of expertise. That was good, right? Plus, she was cheaper than the therapist I'd been seeing for seven years, who was one of the smartest, weirdest healers I'd ever met but still lived in Oakland, where I'd been priced out of. Maybe seeing a therapist in person, not via Skype, would be a good thing? But here I was, in her office, with my mouth open and the rug pulled out from under me.

As it turned out, we had some really different understandings of trauma, healing, and survivorhood. She really thought that childhood sexual abuse was something to manage, something you could get over and "move on" from, a cut you stitch up with butterfly bandages. I thought, *My abuse is not something to resolve, a number on a pain scale, a simple wound that can go away with Neosporin. My trauma is a fucking five-act opera, a gorgeous and tough dress made out of my best scars, a seed library, a Gutenberg Bible, a thunderstorm to climb and buck in a small plane, a mountain range, a supernova to map.*

When I composed myself, I managed to say something like, "I don't really think of it like that—I think that I'm on a lifelong journey of learning from and healing my trauma. You know what I mean?" *You know what I mean, right?*

She smirked at me with that *Poor dear, sure, let her think that* look. And I didn't go back. That therapist wasn't rare. The idea that survivorhood is a thing to "fix" or "cure," to get over, and that the cure is not only possible and easy but the only desirable option, is as common as breath. It's a concept that has deep roots in ableist ideas that when there's something wrong, there's either cured or broken and nothing in between, and certainly nothing valuable in inhabiting a bodymind that's disabled in any way.

It's also an idea that's seductive to survivors. We want the pain, the trauma of surviving sexual abuse or assault to be over. Who wouldn't? What's the problem with that?

Survivorhood is everywhere, yet it's barely spoken about. As I write this essay, the #MeToo movement—a movement encouraging survivors to break our silence and name our survivorhood, first created by Black survivor activist Tarana Burke in 2006, and then Columbused but also re-spread by several white North American actresses and media figures in late 2017, which then took on a life of its own as it was claimed by many everyday survivors who spoke, thought, argued, and organized around survivor issues—has toppled senators and many other famous white men but, more importantly, has created an explosion of survivors telling our stories. The thing I like most about #MeToo is how it, for this media moment, at least, has transformed the experience of being a survivor from one that so often feels freakish and lonely, like I am the only weird one who didn't have a happy, safe family and wants to talk about it, to one where the truth that rape and childhood sexual abuse are the norm, that most people are survivors, is out there.

If you want to argue with me that the CDC and the FBI has said that a mere thirty-three percent of adult assigned-female-at-birth people and twenty-five percent of children are abused, so surely I'm wrong about the "most people are survivors" part, I ask you to consider that I didn't report any of my rapes to the cops and neither do most people I know. There are many forms of sexual abuse, violation, and violence not considered "real rape" by carceral systems—from specific kinds of sexualized abuse that disabled kids face in our families, schools, hospitals, and treatment facilities to ritual abuse, from sexual abuse of Indigenous people in boarding schools and foster care to the constant transmisogynist sexual harassment faced by trans women of color to sexual assault experienced by sex workers. There are new studies that suggest that gender nonconforming children are at greater risk for sexual abuse than cis children—a 2011 study of more than 1,000 transgender people found over fifty percent had experienced sexual violence at some point in our lives, and of those who were adult sexual violence survivors, seventy-two percent had also survived child sexual abuse.[56] Going back to the Black Codes and the Indian Act, the criminal legal system was set up on purpose to minimize what got named as sexual abuse and how much sexual abuse got reported and prosecuted, and limited the tiny percentage of what sexual abuse does get taken seriously to people with less privilege who the system wants to lock up and deport. Throughout my life as a disabled, queer femme of color, I have been surprised when someone I dated or hung out with wasn't a survivor—it was like spotting a unicorn. I've heard tell that it's not much different in straight white land. Denial of abuse's omnipresence—the belief that sexual abuse must be a rarity, happening someplace else by some fundamentally terrible person who looks obviously scary, rather than many violations created by complex, charming, gifted people we know and love, happening right next door—is a big part of what allows childhood and adult sexual abuse to keep going.[57] The latest iteration of #MeToo created space where it's known that the weaponization of sex is not a rarity or an accidental tragedy that befalls a sad handful of people; it's a system of oppression that is in the water and the air. It's also—yes, indeed—expanded the understanding of what rape is to include forms of sexual violation that don't count as "real, classic rape," because survivors are finally having space to voice our own experiences of sex. And although many backlash driven writers decry this, I am incredibly glad for the bravery of survivors expanding the conversation about what sexual abuse and violence are.

---

56   Andrea L. Roberts, Margaret Rosario, Heather L. Corliss, Karestan C. Koenen, and S. Bryn Austin, "Childhood Gender Nonconformity: A Risk Indicator for Childhood Abuse and Posttraumatic Stress in Youth," *American Academy of Pediatrics*, February 2012, http://pediatrics.aappublications.org/content/early/2012/02/15/peds.2011-1804.

57   For some radical perspectives on childhood sexual abuse, check out Generation Five, the Bay Area Transformative Justice Collective, and Mirror Memoirs.

All of this knowledge is dangerous information. If it got out all the way, the world would split open. And it has been, and is. As survivors, we often feel powerless, and we often do lack power—when we can't make an abuser be accountable, when the criminal legal system is racist and whorephobic, when we are the ones who are punished for surviving. But we are also supremely powerful. Our stories of rape and survivorhood are that thundercloud, that nebula. They are huge and awesome, and if they're told, can bring rape culture to its knees.

Rape culture knows this. So it creates many things to manage and suppress survivor knowledge, to tamp it down. The survivor-industrial complex (SIC) is the web of institutions, practices, and beliefs that works to manage, contain, and/or offer resolution to survivors of sexual violence. Its reach is huge, stretching from nurses administering rape kits to YWCA therapists running twelve-week group therapy sessions, from the six-week "solution-focused" therapy that is the only kind available at the sliding scale clinic to the cops and DAs who decide who counts as a "perfect victim" and who's too slutty, poor, Black, brown, crazy, or trans to deserve victim compensation funds. Its management and suppression of survivor truth and rage works much like the nonprofit-industrial complex—which many people work within with the best of intentions, and which was also invented to manage and suppress dissent during the Nixon years.

One of the biggest ways the SIC manages all those messy, powerful survivor emotions and truths is by deploying the idea of the "good" or "fixed" survivor. The "good" survivor is the hypothetical survivor you see on a talk show or a soap opera, who got three months of therapy and is all better: the abuse is a vague memory, there are no visible scars—physical or emotional—and they don't talk about the invisible ones. They have "moved on." They don't talk about the abuse or need access or accommodations about it. They don't bring their abuse into their relationships, jobs, families. They don't bother you with it. This kind of "good" survivor is someone I've never met in person, because they don't exist.

In contrast, the "bad" survivor is the one who is still "broken." Still freaking out, still triggered, still grieving, still remembering. Still making you remember. They're annoying, aren't they? No one wants to date them. They cry, they have panic attacks, they can't get out of bed, they're not "over it." And because of all of that, they're weak, aren't they? They must be weak to not be fixed. All that therapy and they are still not "better"? God. They see the secret inside of the world that is rape culture—every day, ever present and unspoken. They talk about it. "Bad" survivors are mostly absent from pop culture and everyday life yet also ever present—they are the femme with "baggage" you scroll by on Tinder because they look like too much drama, the person who kills themselves who is described later in sorrowful tones as "broken but now at peace," the bitch, the hysteric, the dyke.

The world tells us these stereotypes in a million ways, but we also tell them to ourselves. We torture ourselves with them, and also—let's be real—they're seductive. They make things feel simple. If we believe that some survivors are just too annoying or bitchy, too out of control, we can feel better about ourselves by promising we're not like *that* and distancing ourselves from those bitches.

The promise of cure, of a simple way to be more at peace, that lies inside the "good" survivor is tempting. Of course we want to feel better. As a young survivor, I was in torment every single second of every day, and I wanted not to be. I wanted to fuck. I wanted to stop being so gone from my body that the whole world looked like a TV screen. I wanted to not feel like broken glass. I wanted to be able to think or talk about something other than my incest memories 24-7. I wanted those things because it hurt, and because of the rolled eyes, imagined and real, of the people around me who were impatient at me going on about all that depressing stuff all the time.

There was more. I wanted to interrupt the cycles of abuse and intergenerational violence in my family. I wanted to grow up to have relationships that weren't violent. To know pleasure, not martyrdom. Most of all, I wanted to be happy, and I wanted to know freedom, joy, and liberation. Even though, and especially because, I had no idea what those things actually felt like.

These are powerful, fierce survivor freedom dreams. Dreams like these are where I see many survivors in our fiercest power as revolutionaries. There is revolution in survivors remembering the omnipresence of rape, insisting that we remember shit right, and using our deepest dreams to create new worlds that we have never seen.

There's nothing wrong with wanting less pain, or a different experience of it. There's nothing wrong with wanting to transform generations of passed-down trauma. But what gets more complicated is when those desires bleed into the ableist model of cure that's the only model most of us have for having more ease and less pain. That model and its harsh binary of successful and fixed or broken and fucked is part of what contributes to suicidality and struggle in long-term survivors. I've seen survivors, including myself, struggle with feelings of failure and self-hatred when we're thirty, forty, fifty, sixty, and older and we're still triggered, grieving, and remembering—when we haven't reached that mythic "cured place." In writing this essay, I want to speak to how the thing that keeps me alive and thriving is my work as a disabled survivor to undo pick apart that binary and to name its poison as ableist. To bring together crip and survivor struggles and knowledge. To map a new model of survival where my scars and my still being crazy in adulthood are not signs that I've failed.

CURE, CRIPS, AND SURVIVORS

My friend Blyth Barnow is a white, working-class, femme survivor priest. A couple of months ago, an Instagram photograph she posted blew me away. It was an image of big flip-chart paper in a workshop, with writing that said, *How do survivors' skills translate to ministry?* Underneath, there were words like *boundaries, finding healing moment in texts, nuance, destigmatizing mental health, process of finding healthy self-worth,* and *self-grace.*

Skills. Survivors' skills. Survivors as people who are good at things. Survivors as leaders, because of and not despite our survivorhood. Blyth's post was the first time in my life, after more than twenty years of being deeply integrated in survivor communities, that I'd seen survivors described as being good at things. As having specific skills that emerged from our survivorhood.

There is a deep parallel between the way being a survivor is seen only as a fault, never as a skill, and the way ableism views disabled people as individual, tragic health defects (if you doubt me, think about how disabled fetuses are never referred to as disabled fetuses but as birth defects). When I lead disability justice workshops, one of my toughest teaching moments is always to get people to step out of the deficiency model of disability. When I talk about disabled wisdom and skills, or about disabled people as having histories, cultures, and movements, the blank looks in the room kill me. It's damn near impossible for many abled people to think of disability as anything other than an individual tragedy and a state no one would choose to inhabit.

In the deficiency model of disability, there's nothing good about disability, no skills or brilliance. We are just a fault to be cured. The only good crip is a cured crip, one who has ceased to exist. Cure is healing is elimination.

And cure infects survivor dialogues. Survivors longing for healing hit the medical-industrial complex in search of it, only to confront the idea of cure as the only way to heal from abuse. This belief promotes the binary of fixed or broken, and shame. This binary stops us from being able to imagine survivor futures where we are *thriving* but not *cured.*

When I was a young survivor, I would ask my counselors when "it" would get better, when "it" would be gone. By "it" I meant something between "having flashbacks every day and feeling constantly in trauma land" and "having any trauma memories or experiences at all." I was horrified when one gifted and lovely therapist gently told me that "it" would never fully go away, but my life would and could transform so much I wouldn't even recognize it, and my experience of pain, trauma, and abuse memories would also transform.

My counselor was trying, as best she could, to convey what I would later learn through years of listening to and shape-shifting chronic pain: our experiences of pain and trauma can completely transform when we have access to community, tools, support, and different stories and narratives.

But as that young survivor, the vision I was given from most sources—including some therapists and feminist abuse books—was this: if I performed healing correctly, by the time I was thirty or forty, I would be a survivor who had no visible signs of survivorhood. One who wasn't crazy anymore, who never panicked, never jumped when she was touched the wrong way, who was never brought to her knees by anger or grief or sadness or fear or freezing. The abuse would be gone, and I would be good as new, or as good as someone who had never been abused. It was a vision of survivorhood that mimicked the "good" survivor archetype, albeit with a feminist, anti-oppressive coating.

In this worldview, if I ever had flashbacks, trauma, pain, or triggers, that meant I was failing. At survivorhood. At healing. At fixing it. At "breaking the cycle." This was my life's work, the goal that everything else hung on.

And, then and today, I see survivors struggling with feelings of deep shame that we are not "over it." I see survivors in our thirties, forties, and beyond getting thrown into suicidality when we're triggered, again—not just over the trigger, but because we're beating ourselves up over still being "unfixed." When a new memory or a new experience of trauma or grief comes to us, we think we are failing.

I believe that the answer to these questions lies in bringing a disability justice analysis of ableism into survivor culture. Survivors of sexual or physical abuse who have madness, complex PTSD, multiplicity, or other trauma-rooted psychic differences are part of disability communities. The same skills we have developed as crips, of asking for collective access and resisting ableist ideas, can be a vital part of how we create our reparations and our salvation as survivors.

When we are not fixed, not over it, still triggered, still feeling, still healing in our forties, sixties, and beyond, we are not failing. We are remembering, and we are learning from our survivorhood. We are moving from a model that gasps at our scars to one that wants to learn as much from them as possible. Traditional ideas of survivorhood think of "remembering" as a time-limited process that happens upon recovery of abuse memories and then is over. But in another survivor universe, we are continually expanding—we are always remembering, and remembering again, and thinking about what our wounding means. We are mining our survivor experiences for knowledge.

And I ask the dangerous question: What if more survivors—and the therapists and healing spaces available to us—had a Mad, crip idea of healing, one that was not about cure but about increasing possibility, about learning, about trying to love all our survivor madness, and about shifting our communities to ones where crazy was really okay? What if there were models for long-term grief? Where we had more space in our jobs and homes where it was okay to grieve—like long-term lots of paid grief time off? What would it be like if our communities really, really believed that grief was sacred and valuable, a source of life-giving knowledge, instead of a pain in the ass? What if bad survivors were good survivors? What if all survivors were beautiful in our mess?

And, even more dangerous, I want to venture: What if some things aren't fixable? What if some things really never will be the same—and that might not be great, but it might be okay? I believe in healing and I believe in it happening in ways that are mind-blowing and far beyond what anyone thought possible. But I also wonder, what if some trauma wounds really never will go away—and we might still have great lives? Believing that some things just aren't healable is anathema to most everyone, radical and not. We believe that with enough love and wonderful techniques and prayer, anything can transform. But what if some things can't?

Eli Clare writes about trying to heal his trauma from being tortured and abused by his father:

> Twenty years ago I walked through the world detached from body-mind and emotion, skittish, fearful of human touch, hearing voices and seeing shadows, plotting suicide. When it became clear that I had to deal with this damage or end up dead, all I wanted was to be cured.
>
> I spent years in therapy and bodywork. I practiced self-care and built a support network. I found community. I dug into shame. I helped organize Take Back the Night marches, put together rape prevention trainings, wrote about child abuse. I never spoke directly about my desire for a cure, but really, I felt desperate to fix my broken self, to emerge into a place where the twenty-four years of torture I experienced as a child and young adult simply no longer existed. I spent nearly a decade working hard at recovery—recovering lost years, memories, selves—before I knew that I'd never be cured ... I'm grateful that triggers and hallucinations don't grab me in their vice grip nearly as often as they used to. Even so, I know the past will again

pound through my body-mind ... I've come to know that there will be no cure. I claim brokenness to make this irrevocable shattering visible.[58]

Clare continues, "Cure dismisses resilience, survival, the spider web of fractures, cracks, and seams. Its promise holds power precisely because none of us want to be broken. But I'm curious: what might happen if we were to accept, claim, embrace our brokenness?"

I am curious too. I am curious what might happen if I and we experimented with the dichotomy of fixed or failed. If we let ourselves know that our good, complex, messy, at times painful lives are successes.

At the funeral of our friend Amanda "Arkansassy" Harris, a queer, white, Southern femme photographer who took her life in 2017, Blyth wrote and read a eulogy, "Broken Things," where she talked about the Japanese ceramic art of kintsugi, where a broken vessel is repaired in a way that seeks to emphasize and celebrate the break, rather than hide it. A seam binding two pieces of a cup back together might be filled with a lacquer mixed with gold or another shiny element—a "philosophy not of replacement, but of awe, reverence, and restoration." She said, "For me, there is something very Femme about all of it. The idea that adornment is a form of reverence, of binding together. The notion that our cracks, our wounds, can be beautiful too ... In learning how to heal we have also learned how to mend. We take what is supposed to go unseen and amplify it, make it too much, put gold on it."[59]

I want to put gold all over our old bitch, still-here lives.

---

58   Eli Clare, "Feeling Broken," in *Brilliant Imperfection* (Durham, NC: Duke University Press, 2017), 159–60.

59   Blyth Barnow, "Broken Things: A Eulogy," *Femminary*, February 27, 2017, https://femminary.com/2017/02/27/broken-things-a-eulogy, accessed June 21, 2018.

OLD BITCH SURVIVORS WHO CRY AND LAUGH

As a young survivor, I read a lot of survivor writing—the feminist of color, slam poetry kind, the Dorothy Allison kind. What I picked up on was that telling the raw truth could heal you. Running away could heal you. Cutting off someone's dick could heal you (thank God Lorena Bobbitt was in the news when I was twenty). Sex could heal you, and solitude, and a closed door. Time and space and silence.

What I didn't see much of were stories of what came after—what long-term survivorhood looked like after you'd been trying to heal for a while. Besides the vague encouragement found in *The Courage to Heal* that eventually I'd be a nice normal housewife/social worker who didn't think about my rape much. The two options seemed to be either that or suicide.

It would've meant a lot to me, I think, if I'd seen stories and pictures of some middle-aged or older femme survivors who were happy and yet not done. Who were a lot less triggered than they used to be but still snapped at their partner, froze up when touched a certain way, had a great month and then a panic attack week and then had to just get the fuck out of town for a while. Who were successful on their own terms and who also had at least a few deeply shitty mental health times a year. Who had chosen queer family that was wonderful, the best, and also fell the fuck apart in completely unpredictable ways. Who thought they knew everything about their abuse story, but who then woke up one day at forty-two and thought, *Shit, maybe my mom also abused my older cousin who was like me and who she also had a "special closeness" to,* or, *What if I'm not just grateful to be free; I'm deeply angry and sad that I don't have a mom?* Who had a full rich life, but one where the abuse memories were never faint.

There are still not enough of those stories, so here are some of mine: I'm forty-three and I live in a house with my amazing femme of color partner; a white, disabled, queer artist friend who rents studio space to help out with the rent; and a roommate, plus two cats, in a greenbelt strip in Southside Seattle, where there are big trees and blackberry bushes and a secret creek, and it's also ten minutes from Wendy's. I love my partner, and the survivor, femme of color love I get from them has transformed my heart and my cunt and my life. Living together is amazing and was also super hard in ways I never expected—moving in hit me with all the PTSD from past abuse in the world. Working through all those triggers is real. I love my friends, and I have panic attacks that lay me out for two days that I sometimes still feel deeply ashamed of but am working on it. I'm still unpacking deep shame I have around both "being crazy" and around being the survivor of childhood sexual abuse that is stigmatized (mother-daughter, happened early). By *unpacking* I mean sometimes it hits in a gut punch in the middle of my day, in the middle of negotiating sex or teaching a workshop.

I still feel sad about my abuse. I grieve not having a mom. And I let myself feel fucking sad, because it is fucking sad. Two years ago, my grief about not having a mom hit me right behind the knees the day after Mother's Day, and I stayed there for a long time, and I canceled shit and worked in pajamas and cried longer than I thought there were days and hated it and had no choice. I didn't know that grief was there.

My happiness is messy. It's all of it. I can be defensive and stubborn as hell. I can be wrong. I can have a meltdown. I can be frozen. I can jerk off for hours and not be able to get out of bed. I can win awards. I make dinner for friends. I have somatic flashbacks of my rape. Still. I'm still scared to talk to my family, and visiting the town where I grew up is something I never do casually or without an escape plan. I experience months of joy and weeks that get sucked under when I trip over a wire and a trap door opens. Sometimes I experience deep psychic pain. Sometimes things change.

I have a lot of tools. I have Ativan, prayer, counseling, an altar, DBT cards in my purse, and a shit ton of tinctures and crystals.

Sometimes I grip my steering wheel and have no idea where I am. I perform at Princeton, Hampshire, UC Davis. I am not a supersurvivor or supercrip. I am a crip survivor with superpowers who has joy and sadness, rage and loneliness, grief and discovery.

I don't want to be fixed, if being fixed means being bleached of memory, untaught by what I have learned through this miracle of surviving. My survivorhood is not an individual problem. I want the communion of all of us who have survived, and the knowledge.

I do not want to be fixed. I want to change the world. I want to be alive, awake, grieving, and full of joy. And I am.

CRIP LINEAGES, CRIP FUTURES

A CONVERSATION WITH STACEY MILBERN

Leah: Stacey, remember that thing you posted about crip doulaing on Facebook? It blew my mind. You basically posited this whole new language around crips mentoring and assisting with birthing into disability culture/community, different kinds of disability, etc., as something we already do all the time but there is no language around in abledworld. Say more?

Stacey: Thank you, Leah. I see a lot of disabled people of color doing a ton of work in supporting people rebirthing themselves as disabled (or more disabled). This looks like a lot of things—maybe learning how to get medicine, drive a wheelchair, hire attendants, change a diet, date, have sex, make requests, code switch, live with an intellectual disability, go off meds, etc., etc. The transition itself, of becoming disabled or moving along the ability spectrum, is frequently invisibilized, to the point that these changes do not even have a name. We do not have a way to talk about becoming disabled or more impaired. I feel like society not having language to describe this transition or the support it requires speaks to the ableism and isolation people with disabilities face in our lives. Of course there aren't yet words for this. Without crip intervention, we are frequently left alone to figure out how to be in our bodyminds and in this ableist world.

Crip mentorship/coaching/modeling at its best is "disability doulaship." We—you and I—are doulas. I am thankful for every person who has trusted me with the honor of supporting them through their journey and those who have supported me through the same. My survival and resilience has depended on it.

Leah: Yes. Yes. And that is such a huge paradigm shift—to view coming into disability identity as a birth, not a death, which is how the transition(s) are seen by ableist culture. To see it as a series of births, as our bodyminds evolve in their crip, neurodivergent, Deaf, sick identities over time—to name that there are life stages and rites of passage of becoming disabled, that this is not a static wound, these disabled bodyminds are creative, evolving strategies. Naming disability as a space we can be born into, not alone but supported and welcomed by other disabled people—and then again and again as we acquire new disabilities or discover words for things that have been there all along—that warm doulaed space creates a container that changes not only the entire way both individuals can experience disability but the ways disability communities can be formed.

And crip doulaing is both an interpersonal dynamic and one that creates new disability justice space. My moment where I was like, holy shit, I can actually feel myself a part of a politicized disability community, was around 2007, and I began to find sick and disabled QTBIPOC community around 2008, right? Now, a decade later, I see a younger generation of SDQTBIPOC who both seem to have less struggle talking about ableism as a social justice and lived issue, and who are creating new cultural spaces that blow my mind. The other day, I saw posts by some sick and disabled femmes of color who are creating BDSM parties with detailed access info in houses in Oakland. They're trying to create sexual cultures where discussing trauma, consent, desirability politics, and ableism is a norm, even if it's imperfect and struggling against a violent gentrification real estate market where finding accessible space is challenging. I haven't visited them in person yet, but I'm like, this is light-years ahead of the queer sex cultures I grew up in! (Which so often weren't accessible—not wheelchair or Deaf or fragrance accessible and also just in their assumptions that people have sex and how people have sex.) And I'm like, this happened because of the doulaing as organizing we did, the talking and supporting and hanging out and sharing articles and writing them. Or when I see QWOCMAP (the Queer Women of Color Media Access Project, an annual queer women of color film festival in the Bay Area) have this beautiful, warm, fragrance-free ask on their promotional material, coming from a working-class Black and Asian, middle-aged, partially disabled leadership, framed as being about collective love and support, I think about how some of that being there came from our loving, co-supportive relationships with each other. But I simultaneously am like, GREAT, and also like, is all this history of organizing going to get forgotten in a couple of years, because that's what happens to crip histories period but especially to grassroots, working-class Black, Indigenous, and Brown sick and disabled femme organizing that flies under the radar and is not studied or noticed by abled POC or white crip land? And how do we prevent that from happening? What are our lineages? Who are the crip people and spaces who came before us who we call on, who are often not named in white disabled history?

Stacey: One of the hardest experiences about being disabled QTBIPOC for me is that there is little visibility or acknowledgment we exist, and we are left alone to figure out who we are and where we come from. That struggle to understand and create a genealogy that includes oneself is not necessarily unique to disabled people or queer people of color but nonetheless difficult. We may be the only one like us in our given and chosen family stories. There are so many stories of Deaf people who grow up in hearing families where no one signs. Or I think of my own story. I was the only disabled person in my immediate family, and they loved me but didn't have tools for conceptualizing my life outside of brokenness needing healing or bootstrap mentality about "overcoming" one's circumstance. My heart swells hearing about second- and third-generation families of disabled people, for example, a handful of friends who are people living with dwarfism or Osteogenesis Imperfecta, who are proudly raising kids with dwarfism or OI.

I feel like I have spent lifetimes doing excavation work to find myself and my people, whether it is actively or passively, and most days I don't actually have a lot materially to show for it, except for the poetry of disability justice and relationships with crip queer beloveds. If you are a wheelchair user like myself, especially of color, a woman, a queer person riding gender borders, who are you supposed to see yourself represented in, Franklin D. Roosevelt or the kid from *Glee*? History frequently has not found our lives valuable enough to record-keep or tell our stories, and if it does, the narratives do not look like us, and if they by some miracle chance do, they are riddled with so much ableism that it is hard to separate out how the person with the impairment felt about their life and what is the story keeper's ableist projections onto them.

It is frequently dangerous to seek each other out, even when we are alive in the same time period—disabled people face so much violence on the day to day—and admitting to having an impairment frequently can lead to losing one's parenting rights, bodily autonomy, employment, more. My friends Moya Bailey and India Harville, two Black, queer, disabled activists, and many other people, have done a lot of work to understand how the violent history of subjugation and chattel slavery shapes how Black communities may or may not relate to crip identity and being open about disability when it requires a person to "admit one has a compromised relationship to labor" (Bailey) within a system of ableism that has so often led to isolation, violence, and death.

At the same time, we know disabled people have been surviving, resisting, and leading communities from the beginning of time. We do this work of seeking ourselves out across time and planes, scribbling letters to each other in zines after helping disabled kiddos get through homework, calling out to ancestors while washing dishes, laughing over the ridiculousness of life via text and online groups, documenting our experiences with photos and microblogging, etc., etc. I know, Leah, that you've written about wondering if radical women of color ancestors would have claimed us with all the internalized ableism they faced. It is so hard to know. I wonder frequently what kind of conversation we would have if disability justice activists time-traveled back thirty, forty, fifty years ago and got to share an anti-ableism framework the same time the Combahee River Collective was forming or *This Bridge Called My Back* was penned. What kind of conversations would they have at the kitchen table with us? I want to speculate that the analysis of living in an environment of systemic oppression is functionally what creates disability would resonate with their understanding of intersectionality and oppression. I can also imagine that being open about disability, and some people even being proud of their disability identities, might not translate. That feels understandable, since we needed their work to build these ideas upon.

My own lineage is complicated. It includes my friends who have gone on, disabled friends who might not have politically shared a lot but who so very much wanted to live the life I live now and whom I live in honor of. It includes Korean ancestors I've not gotten yet to know fully. It includes some white disabled women, like Harriet McBryde Johnson and Laura Hershey. Their legacies all are important and a part of me.

Leah: Young abled people are always like, *where are our queer elders?* But it's pretty clear to me where we often are—someplace affordable where we can go to bed early—and what we gain in that move, and also what we lose. My neurodivergent brain and slow body really want some kind of accessible QTBIPOC rural community, but I also get really scared that if I'm not constantly out there as a performer, how fast I'll be forgotten.

We need to ask ourselves, what are the conditions that will allow disabled QTBIPOC elderhood to flourish? For me, some of those conditions are creating accessible community spaces. When I first moved to Oakland, I was struck by how some of the most popular dance nights for queer women of color happened in the afternoon. They were Black and Latinx queer spaces that went from two to eight p.m., they had free (or $5) barbecue and lots of places to sit down. Those spaces had accessibility, even if no one used the word, that made it possible for me to go dancing. And while I was there, I saw women in their fifties and sixties—dancing and hanging out and being able to be part of a queer women of color social world there. When we really value ourselves as queer and trans disabled Black and brown people, the ways our spaces look are going to change—but shit like this proves we already've been doing it! We know how to refuse to forget about each other.

I both do and do not have disabled QTBIPOC elders in my life. Ancestors, yes. Elders, not as much. Elderhood is not a state that just happens. Disabled QTBIPOC elderhood is dependent on systems that support it being there—like affordable rent, neighborhoods that don't gentrify, social spaces that are accessible, Section 8 or social housing that exists and doesn't have a ten-year waiting list, guaranteed annual income, accessible work. When those things don't exist, it affects the likelihood that we'll get to elder.

In the last few years since I turned forty, younger disabled QTBIPOC have started calling me "elder." While I'm honored that they see me as someone they respect and have maybe learned from, it also makes me feel a little desperate. I know that part of why they are naming me as an elder is because I'm the oldest disabled QTBIPOC person they know.

Many sick, disabled, Mad, and neurodivergent older people don't live to get really old. Sometimes that's because of progressive disability, but it's also because of systemic oppression. So many of my sick and disabled QTBIPOC elders are in trailer parks or living in a motel or moved back in with their shitty family because they didn't have a better option. When that class and location slippage happens, they become really invisible to younger hip queers really fucking fast.

Other elders I know have more choices but have withdrawn from the world as they've gotten older, because lack of access doesn't get easier when you get older. In our twenties and thirties, we might have forced ourselves to be visible to abled people, for them to care about us, by organizing and writing and pushing ourselves to be present in abled spaces. But then when we turn forty, we're like, fuck it; we're tired and we can't push ourselves like that in the same way anymore. Often our hearts are broken, or very, very tired, from twenty years of struggle—it really sucks to be having the Access 101 conversation you've been having since the late '80s, again. Our friends are dead, our neighborhood has gentrified, and everyone in the club is twenty-two and has no idea who that old lady/fag/butch is. Our bodyminds never fit that well into capitalism, and as we age we fit into it even less.

What are some moments of birthing ourselves we want to describe?
Stacey: Zora Neale Hurston said there are years that ask questions and years that answer. To be honest, I'm in a year right now of completely being undone. I'm having a hard time with higher levels of daily pain and faster bursts of my progressive neuromuscular disability advancing. I have always had a progressive disability and know what is needed to adjust myself to a big lifestyle change (e.g., becoming less ambulatory in sixth grade, becoming a powerchair user in tenth grade, getting a trach in twelfth grade, etc., etc.), but it is still so hard and painful, and this time it is harder. I find myself having moments where I am closest to all of these edges that I've spent my entire life avoiding—edges of grief, edges of pride or things I thought I'd never

do, edges of shame—and somehow still hanging on, sometimes even dancing on the cliffs. Like the time last week when I was crying in a hospital bed and alone, and instead of having a pity party that none of the chaplains could relate to my experience, the Spirit found me and I preached to myself the words I needed to hear. Or also last week, when I was terrified to be alone after getting out of the ICU—instead of keeping my anxiety to myself and being in terror, I found my mouth telling people that truth (I'm so scared) and asking them to stay and sit, or stay and sleep. I had 24-7 support the first eighty-four hours after the hospital. The sense of being a burden still burns hot in my throat, but the necessity of the moment triumphs. There is nothing more crip than crip practicality. I'm riding an avalanche and won't know how things will land until I crash to a stop. That requires support. A lot of support.

Just as I'm learning to let myself have support and learning to be compassionate with myself, I'm learning to let myself grieve. I let myself go in the low. I give myself a window of time to stay there, and then I come to get me out. I also give myself reality breaks. I spend a lot of my time watching fantasy movies where people transfigure or get to leave their bodies via avatars. I watch them over and over. It's okay that that's my jam. These bodyminds of ours require a lot of us; we can be imperfect, we can cope with shitty things that get us through. I'm thankful for whatever help you get in this life.

Rebirthed me always has new priorities. I let them guide me. This time it's to live life with my disabled love as much as we can with the time and health we have and to let the Spirit transform me through this experience that I may be of use to my communities and people in a way I wasn't before. Everything else forms around those things. Pain and loss clarifies, refines. Sometimes crip life is crystal clear. I know how I want to live in this world. I fight to be here.

How have you found crip ancestors? Do your ancestors feel the same way about disability and ableism as you? What have you learned from them? What are you teaching them?

Leah: I stumbled upon them. I dug them up. I fought to find them. I dreamed them. Others shared them. I remembered them, like oh, the woman who chosen-mothered me when I was eighteen. That was a disabled story because we were two crazy femmes mentoring each other. I think about questions like, what does it mean to claim Marsha P. Johnson and Sylvia Rivera as crip ancestors because they were both chronically ill, trauma-surviving, Mad trans women of color and sex work organizers? What doors open up then in terms of how we understand madness as power, Black and brown trans women's brilliant Mad political actions?

In my own lineage, for years I always said that I became disabled at twenty-two, the first in my family, but as I got older I remembered my mother's story of living with polio—a buried and a fiercely present story, because she closeted her disability to survive, but her pain and physical difference was all up in our house. So often, when we start telling the stories of disability, we realize they are woven into every thread of all our lives.

I don't know if these ancestors feel the same way about disability and ableism as I do. I don't know. Probably not! It's likely they had some wicked internalized ableism and isolation. Or maybe they thought all the same shit I do but it didn't get passed down or recorded/they didn't have anyone to speak it to/no one who cared was listening. Maybe they experienced disability in fundamentally different ways than I did that are not just internalized ableism. I don't know. I am making it up as I go along. I believe running back to look for our disabled ancestors is political work. I believe in sitting in the space of prayer, in the void of not always knowing who is disabled and what their legacy means as a disability justice space. I feel like we are passing knowledge back and forth, beyond the beyond. Being closer to the dead than the living is another kind of crip relationship. I think about the possibilities I am articulating in my life as ones that maybe they were or were not able to embody in their life—but either way, I would not be here without them. Their crip Black and brown queerness gets to breathe because of our storytelling and remembering.

And I wonder, with all our people who have been murdered or died early, this flood of ancestors, are they part of our crip wealth? We mourn our dead, we become our dead, but are our dead also weapons and resources, seed banks?

I also think a lot about crip futurity. It is radical to articulate that we have a past and lineages and cultures, in a world that says we are individual medical defects to be eliminated. AND it is also radical to dream a liberated future by and for sick and disabled, Deaf, neurodivergent, and Mad queer/trans/Black/brown people, for the same reason. Ableism scarcity means we are often feeling like we're just fighting to survive another day, not be buried under erasure or lack of insurance or both—so it is FUCKING HUGE to imagine, what ARE disability justice revolutionary futures? Especially right now, when so many of us are in the throes of being like, here we go, it's early fascism and they're gonna come for the crips first, and none of the abled will notice. Fighting for basic rights—the ACA and ADA not being eliminated, not being warehoused—means often we are panicking and terrified, frozen in reaction. All of that makes it difficult to imagine what we are for, not just what we are against. BUT this is precisely the time when it is the most important for us to imagine a radical disability justice future.

What element does disability justice play in your spiritual life and how does this connect to lineage for you?
Leah: I grew up the kid of lapsed Christians, both of whose families

were forced to convert and faced a lot of violence in Christian spaces. They left but still retained a lot of scars from the Christianity they knew, and I wanted something else. As a survivor kid, I found solace and connected with spirit in running away to the woods and talking to the moon. And as I got older, I learned a lot about earth-based and ancestor-loving spirituality from multiple traditions, from library books about Wicca to other QTBIPOC friends who talked about ancestors and ways as South Asians we were trying to reconnect to our spiritual traditions without casteism, patriarchy, or Hindutva.

So I have crip ancestors on my altar, and I pray for them and to them. I ask them to help me—to help me figure out how to write something, be in right relation, deal with a problem or conflict in community, survive, deal with my having to interface with the medical-industrial complex. Right now, the people up there include Baba Ibrahim Abdurrahman Farajajé, Leslie Feinberg, Taueret Davies, Galvarino, Gloria Anzaldúa, Frida Kahlo, Audre Lorde, Emma Deboncoeur. They remind me that we are and have been here and heroic in complex ways; we have survived crazy shit and done crazy shit, dealt with complex questions, and not always had all the answers. They remind me that I come from somewhere, that we are not the first people to do DJ work, and that we get to do meaningful things as imperfect people. Too often, people in social justice spaces pedestalize ancestors as saints, and I think it's important to resist that. Disabled ancestors' crip ideas of ancestry, because concepts of perfection are ableist and we sure aren't "perfect!" And we're still valuable.

Stacey: I grew up evangelical Christian in the American South. I was all in ... My parents took me to every healing service in the Carolinas (there are televangelist Benny Hinn videos with me on them). I taught Sunday school, and I was totally the nerd organizing prayer events at school. It really impacted my sense of self to hear that I was broken and unlovable by God because I was disabled and, then later, queer.

Some people legit thought I was disabled because of some sin my mom must have done. I stopped being the same kind of Christian as my parents when church bullies told me I hadn't been healed by God yet because I "didn't believe enough." We were all thirteen years old.

I have done a lot of work on my faith and, surprisingly, have come back to believing in God. My faith is a huge part of my resiliency practice because it answers a lot of my questions. I know disabled people are perfect as we are because I believe we were made by the same hand that made flowers, and mice and dogs and stars, and they are perfect as they are. I know God wants us to strive for justice because God is love and "justice is what Love looks like in public" (Cornel West). I don't know why suffering happens, but I know it hurts God, and I feel the Divine's presence with me through loves who join me in the hard moments.

What does crip wealth mean to you?
Leah: I always go to generosity, and "crip kindness." Crip kindness is the wealth and skill where we notice each other's pain face and offer a chair, ask in a low-key way if we can help with a service task, sit without speaking, drop a bottle of tincture next to someone having a panic attack, raise thousands of dollars for someone to buy an accessible van, or mail a stranger our extra prescription. It's collective noticing and collective hustle. It's being witnessed. It's being allowed to relax, expand, just be.

It's also not automatic, which is a place where I want to deepen Mia Mingus's idea of "access intimacy." Like many other sick and disabled queers, Mia's well-known essay "Access Intimacy" has been foundational to my disability justice knowledge in its naming the experience of crip-on-crip understanding of each other's access needs as a place of love and communion. But some of that essay reads to me like understanding each other's access needs is an automatic and magical process. I want to push back on that and say that while access intimacy is often a sophisticated disabled gift, and we are magic and make magic, I want to argue for access intimacy as a process and a learnable skill. I think it's dangerous when we believe that as disabled people we always "just know" each other's needs—I want us to acknowledge the ways that crips do have ways of knowing each other's "stuff" and how we also need to not assume and ask each other what our needs are. I also think it's very important to state that abled people can and do commit to learning access intimacy, through asking and respecting our knowledge—because otherwise we'll be stuck in this place where we're the only ones who can do for us. I want *everyone* to have crip knowledge.

Crip wealth is also the gift of us being the normal. The gift of, yes, you can live in your sweatpants, you can change your ostomy bag in front of me, you can be really, really weird, the amount of time it takes for you to transfer to the toilet is normal. I see so many abled people running into disability or madness or illness and just being completely flummoxed by all of this, because the ableist shame everyone swims in is so deep. Not that I have shame beat—this is something that I've seen get thrown at us sometimes, "Oh, I'm not like you totally shame-free DJ people"—but I totally still grapple with shame all the time. But some of our wealth is creating these small spaces away from shame, where it is okay to have a disabled bodymind.

Stacey: Leah, this concept you introduced me to has totally been a paradigm shifter! Crip wealth. I'm not going to go into defining it but want to say that I feel like even thinking about crip wealth is so crip itself. I see disabled people every day thinking of ideas abled people never would have, primarily by focusing their time and efforts on using what they do have, and the space between, rather than putting their attention on the limitation or lack of ability. It sounds a little like inspiration porn, but we do come up with wildly imaginative solutions this way. I can ramp a three-inch step by taking off my sneakers and rolling over them. I've seen blind friends do wicked things with text to speech in their ear. My friend Leroy Moore taught me that one way Harriet Tubman was able to scout so many routes is by using her traumatic brain injury and talking aloud to herself; people brushed her off as a crazy woman. Texting, now used by everyone, was created as assistive technology for Deaf people. I save so much time sometimes letting strangers in public assume I can't speak. We have so much at our disposal and most of the world has no idea. It can give us a big toolbox to play with.

What haunts you about ableism?
Leah: Shit, Stacey. Thank you for using the word "haunted." I wouldn't have, but that word captures the ghosts and grief of ableism that haunt me, the corridors of my mind in the nights.

So much haunts me. I have so much crip grief around abled BIPOC organizing that cares about disability and ableism for a year or a few months or a season and then just ... forgets about it. I live in a city, Seattle, right now, where people go, OMG, that is heaven for SDQTPOC! and I'm like, laughing because what they think of as this "big disability justice scene" is like twenty people! Despite there having been disabled activism by people like Billie Rain, E.T. Russian, and many others here for decades, there's still a huge gap where abled queers are just like, *what?* We're the ghosts where they wonder where we went, or they don't even wonder, they just think of us fleetingly now and then but don't hold enough cripworld knowledge to maintain relationships with us—which would mean making systematic change in how they run their lives and gathering spaces.

I am haunted by how I am forgotten by non-disabled activists of color. How most people won't give up the points and success they get from moving in abled time to be with us meaningfully. They'll do lip service about sustainability, but that's it. They will point at the three years disabled people were able to organize in a space they created as how committed they are to anti-ableism but erase the way they stopped supporting us that didn't allow us to continue.

There's also crip bitterness—something very few abled people understand that works to isolate us, because they can't deal with how "harsh" or "depressing" we are to be around and quietly stop working with us. The lack of understanding of the wear and tear of having to be stuck fighting for basic access after twenty-five years of work.

I am haunted by the question of, will all our work and lives be remembered and by who and how? Most DJ folks I know are really nervous about our work being co-opted and ripped off, for good reason, and I'm worried about that too, but I'm equally worried about us being deliberately erased. I believe that our work often thrives in the small scale, the ignored, the underground. I thrive in those cracks myself. But I want disabled QTBIPOC to find each other, find our work, our paradigms, our tools, our science, our hacks and art and love, and it just takes one huge personal relationship fallout to make a community inaccessible or erase years of work. There is no disability justice archive yet. (Another thing to work on.) I remind myself we are each other's archive. Anytime an SD person remembers each other and moments in movement history, we memorialize our history, we witness ourselves into being.

Finally, I am haunted by my dead. The first queer love I had was another suicidal femme, and I have loved Crazy femmes all my life, romantically, sexually, as friends. Many of them are not here anymore. I was organizing my storage closet yesterday and started to sift through my archives—all these piles of papers, zines, cards, event promo cards, of twenty years of QTBIPOC organizing—and when I said online, wow, 2010 sure was different, and someone asked me to explain, one of my first thoughts was of how many more people were alive then. I am haunted by the fact that I will continue to lose femmes I love, as much as I will fight to create and share tools that could help us stay here.

Stacey: I feel heavy with the weight of our longing. Sometimes it haunts me. All of the dreams of our ancestors, disabled people currently living, and disabled people to come. There is so much I want for us, that we want for ourselves and each other. Every person I ever met in an institution, a day program, a sheltered workshop, on the street, on the bus, anywhere has wanted and deserved so much that the world has not given. I feel immense privilege and responsibility for everything I have access to, and it haunts me how many disabled people do not share the same access, even to basic things like a person to talk to who cares about you or choosing the place you live, what you wear, eat, who puts their hands on your body, etc. When I first moved to the Bay, I had a lot of survivor's guilt. The life I was getting to live that loved ones I knew wanted and deserved just as equally but did not have.

Have you thought what you want your legacy to be? How have you held envisioning future, navigating trauma of past, surviving the present all at the same time?

Leah: Oh Christ, I don't know. Yes. Yes, I have thought about it. I write my obituary in my head often. I want to be remembered as the person who broke the cycle of abuse in my family. I want the messy, real, concrete ways I made this happen to be remembered, as one of many possibility models for ending abuse. I want to be remembered as a writer, storytelling performer, and grassroots intellectual—that by telling stories I helped change the world. I want the fragile and strong spaces where we came together as disabled BIPOC, the doorways coming and going, to be remembered. I want to be remembered as one of the many who hung out and lay down and laughed and texted each other ideas and did medical advocacy and did not forget each other and changed the world. Small and big changes that I pray will make a disability justice future. I want to be remembered as that femme cane dancing with you in your chair in the club, or hanging out on our couch plotting and laughing.

Stacey: I want my legacy to be loving disabled people. It has been my life story and work. Through loving disabled people, I get to love myself.

FURTHER READING AND RESOURCES

DISABILITY JUSTICE

Alland, Sandra, Khairani Barokka, and Daniel Sluman, eds. *Stairs and Whispers: D/deaf and Disabled Poets Write Back*. Rugby, UK: Nine Arches Press, 2017.

Autistic Hoya. https://www.autistichoya.com.

Autistic Self Advocacy Network. http://autisticadvocacy.org.

Autistic Self Advocacy Network, "Autism and Safety Toolkit: Safety Tips for Self-Advocates." https://autisticadvocacy.org/wp-content/uploads/2017/11/Autism-and-Safety-Pt-2.pdf, 2018.

Bailey, Moya. "Race and Disability in the Academy." *Sociological Review*. November 8, 2017. https://www.thesociologicalreview.com/blog/race-and-disability-in-the-academy.html.

Ben-Moshe, Liat, Chris Chapman, and Allison C. Carey, eds. *Disability Incarcerated: Imprisonment and Disability in the United States and Canada*. New York: Palgrave Macmillan, 2014.

Bianco, Neve. "My Apparatus." *Model View Culture*. September 8, 2014. https://modelviewculture.com/pieces/my-apparatus.

The Body Is Not an Apology. https://thebodyisnotanapology.com/.

Brown, Lydia X. Z., E. Ashkenazy, and Morénike Giwa Onaiwu, eds. *All the Weight of Our Dreams: On Living Racialized Autism*. DragonBee Press, 2017.

Brown, Lydia X. Z., Leroy Moore, and Tallia Lewis. "Accountable Reporting on Disability, Race, & Police Violence: A Community Response to the 'Ruderman White Paper on the Media Coverage of Use of Force and Disability." https://docs.google.com/document/d/117eoVeJVP594L6-1bgL8zpZrzgojfsveJwcWuHpkNcs/edit?usp=sharing.

Canaries, http://wearecanaries.com/tag/carolyn-lazard/.

Clare, Eli. *Brilliant Imperfection: Grappling with Cure*. Durham, NC: Duke University Press, 2017.

———. *Exile and Pride: Disability, Queerness, and Liberation*. Durham, NC: Duke University Press, 2015.

The Deaf Poets Society. https://www.deafpoetssociety.com/.

"Disability and Access Toolkit." Showing Up for Racial Justice. http://nb.showingupforracialjustice.org/disability_access_toolkit.

"Disability Solidarity: Completing the 'Vision for Black Lives.'" *Harriet Tubman Collective*. https://harriettubmancollective.tumblr.com/post/150072319030/htcvision4blacklives.

Disability Visibility Project, https://disabilityvisibilityproject.com.

Donovan, Colin, and Qwo-Li Driskill, eds. *Scars Tell Stories: A Queer and Trans (Dis)ability Zine*. Seattle: RESYST, 2007.

Driskill, Qwo-Li. *Walking with Ghosts: Poems*. Cromer, UK: Salt Publishing, 2005.

Ejiogu, N., and Syrus Marcus Ware. "How Disability Studies Stays White and What Kind of White It Stays." New York: Society for Disability Studies Conference, City University of New York, 2008.

Eminism.org, http://eminism.org/.

Hershey, Laura, *Spark Before Dark*. Finishing Line Press, 2011.

Johnson, Cyree Jarelle. "Black Cripples Are Your Comrades, Not Your Counterpoint." *Huffington Post*. February 2, 2017. https://www.huffingtonpost.com/entry/black-cripples-your-comrades-not-counterpoint_us_589dbb37e4b094a129ea32b8.

———. *Slingshot*. New York: Nightboat Books, 2019.

Kafer, Allison, *Feminist, Queer, Crip*. Bloomington, IN: Indiana University Press, 2013.

Kaufman, Miriam, Cory Silverberg, and Fran Odette. *The Ultimate Guide to Sex and Disability: For All of Us Who Live with Disabilities, Chronic Pain, and Illness*. San Francisco: Cleis, 2003.

Kim, Eunjung. *Curative Violence: Rehabilitating Disability, Gender, and Sexuality in Modern Korea*. Durham: Duke University Press, 2017.

Koyama, Emi, with Adrie. "Adrie's Guide to Service Animal: Laws, Rights, and Maneuvers for People Living with Disabilities." Portland, OR: Confluere Publications, 2015. http://www.confluere.com/store/pdf-zn/serviceanimals.pdf.

Lazard, Carolyn. "How to Be a Person in the Age of Autoimmunity." https://static1.squarespace.com/static/55c40d69e4b0a45eb985d566/t/58cebc9dc534a59fbdbf98c2/1489943709737/Howtobe aPersonintheAgeofAutoimmunity+%281%29.pdf.

Lorde, Audre. *A Burst of Light*. Mineola, NY: Ixia Press, 2017 (first printing, 1988).

———. *The Cancer Journals: Special Edition*. San Francisco: Aunt Lute Books, 2006.

Lowe, J.S.A. "How to Be Seriously Mentally Interesting: A Primer for Beginners." *Medium*. July 25, 2015. https://medium.com/@jsalowe/how-to-be-seriously-mentally-interesting-a-primer-for-beginners-d1b22490ac65.

M., Bri. *Power Not Pity* podcast. http://www.powernotpity.com.

Milbern, Stacey and Patty Berne, with Dean Spade. "Ableism Is the Bane of My Motherfucking Existence," "My Body Doesn't Oppress Me, Society Does," and "The Ability to Live: What Trump's Health Cuts Mean for People with Disabilities." Part of the No Body Is Disposable series by the Barnard Center for Research on Women, May 25, 2017. https://vimeo.com/218963640.

Mingus, Mia. "Access Intimacy, Interdependence and Disability Justice." *Leaving Evidence*. April 12, 2017. https://leavingevidence.wordpress.com/2017/04/12/access-intimacy-interdependence-and-disability-justice/.

———. "Changing the Framework: Disability Justice." *Leaving Evidence*. February 12, 2011. https://leavingevidence.wordpress.com/2011/02/12/changing-the-framework-disability-justice/.

Moore Jr., Leroy Franklin. *Black Kripple Delivers Poetry & Lyrics*. Lake Isabella, CA: Poetic Matrix Press, 2015.

Morales, Aurora Levins. *Kindling: Writings on the Body*. Cambridge, MA: Palabrera Press, 2013.

———. *Medicine Stories*. Revised edition. Durham, NC: Duke University Press, 2018.

Ndopu, Eddie. "Decolonizing My Body, My Being." The Feminist Wire, December 2012, http://thefeministwire.com/2012/12/a-photo-essay-decolonizing-my-body-my-being/.

People of Color and Mixed-Race Caucus. "Statement of the People of Color and Mixed-Race Caucus from the Queer Disability Conference, 2002." http://www.billierain.com/wp-content/uploads/2010/02/queer-disability-POC-.pdf.

Radical Access Mapping Project. https://radicalaccessiblecommunities.wordpress.com.

Rain, Billie. "Class Disability and Social Darwinism." *The Billie Rain Show*. February 2, 2013. http://www.billierain.com/2013/02/06/class-disability-and-social-darwinism/.

Russian, E.T. *The Ring of Fire Anthology*. Seattle: Left Bank Books, 2014.

Sins Invalid. "Access Suggestions for a Public Event." January 24, 2017. http://sinsinvalid.org/blog/access-suggestions-for-a-public-event.

———. "Access Suggestions for Mobilizations." January 24, 2017. http://sinsinvalid.org/blog/access-suggestions-for-mobilizations.

———. *Sins Invalid: An Unashamed Claim to Beauty*. New Day Films, 2013.

———. *Skin, Tooth, and Bone: The Basis of Movement Is Our People: A Disability Justice Primer*. Available from info@sinsinvalid.org.

Solomon, Rivers. *An Unkindness of Ghosts*. New York: Akashic, 2017.

Taylor, Kara, and Jennie Duguay. "Can Broken Be Whole?" *GUTS*, no. 7 (November 2016). http://gutsmagazine.ca/broken/.

Tovah. "Crip Lit: Towards an Intersectional Crip Syllabus." *Autostraddle*. May 23, 2016. https://www.autostraddle.com/crip-lit-an-intersectional-queer-crip-syllabus-333400/.

"26 Ways to Be in the Struggle—Beyond the Streets." *Tikkun Daily*. December 18, 2014. http://www.tikkun.org/tikkundaily/2014/12/18/26-ways-to-be-in-the-struggle-for-liberation-beyond-the-streets/.

Ware, Syrus Marcus, Joan Ruzsa, and Giselle Dias. "It Can't Be Fixed Because It's Not Broken: Racism and Disability in the Prison Industrial Complex." In *Disability Incarcerated: Imprisonment and Disability in the United States and Canada*, edited by Liat Ben-Moshe, Chris Chapman, Allison C. Carey. New York: Palgrave Macmillan, 2014.

Wear Your Voice. https://wearyourvoicemag.com.

When Language Runs Dry: A Zine for People with Chronic Pain and Their Allies. http://chronicpainzine.blogspot.com.

Wong, Alice. *Resistance and Hope: Essays by Disabled People*. Disability Visibility Project, 2018.

EMOTIONAL LABOR

Hoffman, Ada. "Autism and Emotional Labour." January 30, 2018. http://www.ada-hoffmann.com/2018/01/30/autism-and-emotional-labour/.

Morrigan, Clementine. "Three Thoughts on Emotional Labor." *GUTS*. June 12, 2017. http://gutsmagazine.ca/emotional-labour/.

Thom, Kai Cheng. "8 Lessons That Show How Emotional Labor Defines Women's Lives. *Everyday Feminism*. June 15, 2016. http://everydayfeminism.com/2016/06/emotional-labor-womens-lives/.

Weiss, Suzannah. "50 Ways People Expect Constant Emotional Labor from Women and Femmes." *The Body Is Not an Apology*. January 28, 2018. https://thebodyisnotanapology.com/magazine/50-ways-people-expect-constant-emotional-labor-from-women-and-femmes/.

Willes, Brett Cassady. "Femme Kinship Is Magic." *GUTS*. January 13, 2017. http://gutsmagazine.ca/femme-kinship-is-magic/.

SUICIDE AND SERIOUSLY MENTALLY INTERESTING RESOURCES

Bornstein, Kate. *Hello, Cruel World! 101 Alternatives to Suicide for Teens, Freaks and Other Outlaws.* New York: Seven Stories Press, 2006.

Directory of Crisis Respite Houses. https://power2u.org/directory-of-peer-respites/.

Icarus Project Crisis Toolkit. http://theicarusproject.net/welcome-to-the-crisis-toolkit/.

Monster Academy. https://monsteracademymtl.wordpress.com.

National Queer & Trans Therapists of Color Database. http://www.nqttcn.com/.

Thom, Kai Cheng. "8 Tips for Trans Women of Color Who Are Considering Suicide." Everyday Feminism. November 7, 2015. http://everydayfeminism.com/2015/11/for-trans-women-considering-suicide/.

———. "Stop Letting Trans Girls Kill Ourselves." *Who Will Walk These Wooden Streets?* November 2, 2016. http://sintrayda.tumblr.com/post/152630841778/stop-letting-trans-girls-kill-ourselves-not-a.

Trans Lifeline. (Staff will not call the cops no matter what, is for trans and gender nonconforming folks and friends/allies, voice and text.) https://www.translifeline.org/, 877-565-8860.

Wright, Cortez. "Learning to Live with Wanting to Die." This Body Is Not an Apology. June 10, 2018. http://thebodyisnotanapology.com/magazine/learning-to-live-with-wanting-to-die/.

A BUNCH OF BLACK, QUEER, FEMME-CREATED RESOURCES, PROVIDING SHORT-TERM, IN-THE-MOMENT BODY-BASED WAYS TO HELP HOLD GRIEF, TRAUMA, AND CRISIS

"Care for Ourselves as Political Warfare." http://adriennemareebrown.net/2014/12/10/caring-for-ourselves-as-political-warfare/.

"Just Healing Resources." https://justhealing.wordpress.com/resourcing-the-work/.

"Survival Tips for Radical Empaths." http://adriennemareebrown
.net/2016/11/10/survival-tips-for-radical-empaths/.

CHEMICAL INJURY AND FRAGRANCE ACCESS

"Fragrance-Free Femme of Color Genius." https://www.brownstargirl
.org/blog/fragrance-free-femme-of-colour-realness-draft-15.

"MCS Accessibility Basics." http://www.billierain.com/2011/03/12/
mcs-accessibility-basics/.

"3 Steps to Organizing a Fragrance-Free Event." http://www.billierain
.com/2011/05/01/3-steps-to-organizing-a-fragrance-free-event/.

HEALING JUSTICE

Bad Ass Visionary Healers. https://badassvisionaryhealers.wordpress.com/.

Harriet's Apothecary. http://www.harrietsapothecary.com.

Just Healing. https://justhealing.wordpress.com/.

Midnight Apothecary. http://midnightapothecary.blogspot.com/.

Midnight, Dori. "More Healing, More of the Time." *Midnight Apothecary.*
October 17, 2012. http://midnightapothecary.blogspot.com/2012/10/
more-healing-more-of-time.html.

Padamsee, Yashna Maya. "Communities of Care, Organizations for
Liberation." *Naya Maya.* June 19, 2011. https://nayamaya.wordpress.
com/2011/06/19/communities-of-care-organizations-for-liberation/.

Page, Cara. "Reflections from Detroit: Transforming Wellness &
Wholeness." June 2010. https://inciteblog.wordpress.com/2010/08/05/
reflections-from-detroit-transforming-wellness-wholeness/.

Raffo, Susan. "The Medical Industrial Complex with Gratitude to Mia
Mingus, Patty Berne and Cara Page (Plus Others)." November 28,
2017. http://susanraffo.blogspot.com/2017/11/the-medical-industrial-
complex-with.html.

Third Root. https://thirdroot.org/.

Werning, Kate. *Healing Justice* podcast. https://www.healingjustice.org.

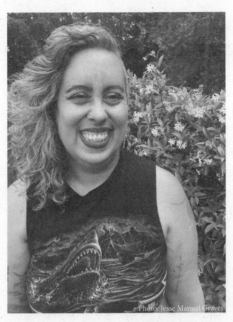
Photo: Jesse Manuel Graves

LEAH LAKSHMI PIEPZNA-SAMARASINHA is a queer disabled femme writer, organizer, performance artist, and educator of Burgher/Tamil Sri Lankan and Irish/Roma ascent. They are the author of the memoir *Dirty River: A Queer Femme of Color Dreaming Her Way Home* (short-listed for the Lambda and Publishing Triangle Awards), and the poetry collections *Bodymap, Love Cake* (Lambda Literary Award winner), and *Consensual Genocide*, and coeditor of *The Revolution Starts at Home: Confronting Intimate Violence in Activist Communities*. Their next two books, *Tonguebreaker* and *Exploring Transformative Justice: A Reader* (coedited with Ejeris Dixon), are forthcoming in 2019. A lead artist with Sins Invalid, her writing has been widely anthologized, and she speaks and perform at universities, conferences, and community events across North America. She is a VONA Fellow and holds an MFA from Mills College.

brownstargirl.org